LIVING
POSITIVELY
IN A WORLD
WITH HIV/AIDS

LIVING
POSITIVELY
IN A WORLD
WITH HIV/AIDS

MARK de SOLLA PRICE

AVON BOOKS ◆ NEW YORK

"Love Don't Need A Reason (An HIV/AIDS Anthem)" by Peter Allen, Michael Callen, and Marsha Malamet reprinted by permission of the Estate of Michael Callen.

LIVING POSITIVELY IN A WORLD WITH HIV/AIDS is an original publication of Avon Books. This work has never before appeared in book form.

AVON BOOKS
A division of
The Hearst Corporation
1350 Avenue of the Americas
New York, New York 10019

Copyright © 1995 by Metamorphics Corporation
Interior text design by Suzanne H. Holt
Published by arrangement with Metamorphics Corporation
Library of Congress Catalog Card Number: 94-16832
ISBN: 0-380-77623-5

Library of Congress Cataloging in Publication Data:
Price, Mark de Solla, 1960–
   Living positively in a world with HIV/AIDS / Mark de Solla Price.
      p.   cm.
Includes bibliographical references.
1. AIDS (Disease)—Popular works.   I. Title.
RC607.A26D4   1995   94-16832
362.1'969792—dc20   CIP

First Avon Books Trade Printing: May 1995

AVON TRADEMARK REG. U.S. PAT. OFF. AND IN OTHER COUNTRIES, MARCA REGISTRADA, HECHO EN U.S.A.

Printed in the U.S.A.

OPM   10   9   8   7   6   5   4   3   2

DEDICATION

Living Positively in a World with HIV/AIDS is dedicated to my dear friend and companion, Vinny Allegrini; my late mother, Ellen de Solla Price (1925–1995); and my wonderful family, Linda, Jeff, and Nancy, and their children, Eva, Aaron, Thomas, and Becky.

It is these people, most of all, who have taught me what unconditional love is all about, and what it means to live positively.

This book is also dedicated to the forty million or so people worldwide who will have had to live with HIV/AIDS by the year 2000, with the hope that perhaps some of what we have learned from the hundreds of thousands of Americans who have already died will help those still living to improve the quality and quantity of their lives.

Love Don't Need A Reason
(An HIV/AIDS Anthem)

If your heart always did, what a normal heart should do. If you always play a part instead of being who you really are, then you might just miss the one who's standing there.

So instead of passing by, show him that you care. Instead of asking why? Why me? And why you? Why not we two?

'Cause love don't need a reason. Love don't always rhyme. And love is all we have for now. What we don't have is time.

If we always believe all the madness that we're taught. Never questioning the rules, then we're living lies we bought so long ago. How are they to know?

It's not who's wrong or right, it's just another way. And I don't wanna fight, but know I'm gonna stay with you till the end. With you my friend.

'Cause love don't need a reason. Love don't always rhyme. And love is all we have for now. What we don't have is time.

I'll hold you close. Time can't tear us apart. Forever, I will stand by you. We've got to start with the beat of two hearts. Together, we will see this through.

'Cause love don't need a reason. Love's never a crime. And love is all we have for now. What we don't have, what we don't have, is time.

—PETER ALLEN
(1944–1992)
—MICHAEL CALLEN
(1955–1993)
—MARSHA MALAMET

CONTENTS

ABOUT THE TERM "HIV/AIDS"

Some people may be surprised to read that there continues to be a great deal of controversy over what the exact definition of "AIDS" should be, what alternative names might be more appropriate, and exactly what the factor (or factors) that causes AIDS should be named.

These are all certainly important issues, and are discussed in greater detail in this book. But it is important to remember that these are, in the end, only words.

In this book, we want to get beyond the words, to actions and attitudes that help improve the quality and quantity of life for those dealing with these issues, whatever they are called. I have chosen to use "HIV/AIDS" consistently throughout the book because it will be understood by the largest possible audience.

It is my hope that those who are so well informed that they feel uncomfortable with some of the limitations in this wording will be able to understand why it was necessary and will read beyond it.

INTRODUCTION

I wrote this book for many reasons, but most of all I wrote it because it was the book I most needed to read. Living with HIV/AIDS is rarely easy, and I needed to remind myself of some of the wonderful things I have learned along the way. It also became too painful for me not to write this book. The idea that all this great wisdom I encountered might get lost and be forgotten was just too depressing. I hope that it doesn't lose too much in my retelling.

This is not a book of "musts" or "shoulds." These are only options and alternatives, tools and techniques. Think of them as the suggestions for the buffet of life. Just because I love *crème brûlée* and hate *soft-shelled crab* doesn't mean that you should make the same choices.

> *Too much of a good thing can be wonderful.*
> —*MAE WEST*

The making of this book began perhaps fifteen years ago, way back in The Disco Era of the late 1970s and early 1980s. It was a magical time filled with glitter and glamour. I was lucky to have been the right age, at the right time, and in the right place. I worked (and played) at the very center of it all, in New York's legendary entertainment and media industry. Discotheques such as Studio 54, Palladium, AREA and The Saint were the place for everyone—from billionaires to busboys, from senators' wives to salesclerks—to see and be obscene.

Unfortunately, this also happened to be the exact

time and place that was first affected by the AIDS epidemic.

Looking back from today's "just-say-no" morality, it's strange to remember there was once a time, not too long ago, when we all looked at things a little differently. American technology multinationals like Dow Chemical promised the whole world "better living through chemistry."

For my generation, this took on a new meaning: We "improved" upon nature with chemical pesticides, fertilizers, food additives, and ultraprocessing. Cigarettes, marijuana, and even cocaine were "proven" harmless and considered to be as nonaddictive as vitamins.

Casual sex of any description with anyone in tight jeans was very fashionable back then. All of the indulgences that we're prone to at the close of the twentieth century were considered just good, clean, healthy fun. This is very different from the way things are now—although many people still do these things, it's not socially acceptable to talk about them anymore.

In the more than dozen years since then, every day I have lived in a world with HIV/AIDS. I think I understand how the few who survived Hiroshima or the Warsaw Ghetto must have felt. Over the years I have scratched over one hundred names out of my address book, and the world I once knew simply doesn't exist anymore.

Those early years were the roughest. We were all so afraid. There were no effective medical treatments and very little hope. The press had labeled it the "gay cancer," and well-meaning health officials moralized at us.

It's like living in wartime. The first casualties were mostly men in their twenties and thirties, filled with promise and excitement. It's easy for me to get stuck looking back nostalgically at old photo albums of friends "I Remember." But this is the past and,

One has to be beyond sex one day, but the way beyond goes through it, and if you never go into it rightly, it is very difficult to go beyond it. So going through it is part of going beyond.

—BHAGWAN SHREE RAJNEESH

frankly, much of it did need changing.

Now is the time for us to move on and reinvent our future. We must turn this catastrophic heartbreak into an opportunity to rebuild ourselves—as a community, as a country, and a world—into something better than we were before.

Slowly, the public is starting to realize that HIV/AIDS is everyone's business. Magic Johnson has helped. Mary Fisher, Ryan White, Arthur Ashe, Allison Gertz, Rock Hudson, and Congressman Stewart McKinney have all helped. But millions of people need more information. A lot more information.

It's my hope that *Living Positively in a World with HIV/AIDS* will help people to understand that HIV/AIDS can be viewed as a treatable, chronic condition you can learn to live with, and that it can be a wake-up call to start living life to the fullest—as it has been for so many.

The music of this opera (Madam Butterfly) was dictated to me by God; I was merely instrumental in putting it on paper and communicating it to the public.
— *GIACOMO PUCCINI*

Naturally, a book like this cannot be written by one person alone. I would like to offer my special thanks to John Thompson, Steven M. Price, Jeffrey Price, Cathy Parsons, Linda DeMichele, John Jones, Albert ten Brink, Dr. Ron Grossman, Marianne Williamson, Fred Small, Sean Strub, Fran Peavey, Maureen Owen, and Pam Meier for their generous help and support for this project.

I would like to thank Ava Lev, Samuel Kirshner, Gay Men's Health Crisis, the Healing Circle, Manhattan Center for Living, Friends In Deed, and the anonymous members of twelve-step fellowships and support groups for their help, understanding, and wisdom.

This project could never have been dreamed of if it weren't for my remarkable tenth-grade English teacher at Choate, Harriet Johnson, who showed me all those years ago that I could write. She broke all the rules to help me understand that having dyslexia and a D average in English did not prevent me from writing something worthwhile.

The ideas I stand for are not mine. I borrowed them from Socrates. I swiped them from Chesterfield. I stole them from Jesus. And I put them in a book. If you don't like their rules, whose would you use?

—DALE CARNEGIE

I would also like to thank my wonderful agent, Nancy Love; and Lisa Considine, Rachel Klayman, Bob Mecoy, David Highfill, Sara Schwager, and Matthew Sartwell from Avon Books for the opportunity to bring this work to such a wide audience.

I would like to thank the following people for their inspirational work, upon which everything I have done is based: Bernie S. Siegel; Louise Hay; Benjamin Hoff; David Keirsey; Derek Humphry; Elisabeth Kübler-Ross; Graham Kerr; George R. Melton; Gerald Jampolsky; Gerald M. Weinberg; John Bradshaw; John-Roger; Larry Kramer; M. Scott Peck; Marilyn Bates; Michael Callen; Nick Siano; Norman Cousins; Pat Califia; Paul Monette; Perry Tilleraas; Peter McWilliams; Peter Tatchell; Randy Shilts; Richard Nelson Bolles; Ryan White; Shakti Gawain; Sogyal Rinpoche; Stephen Levine; and Wally Amos.

—Mark de Solla Price
May 1995
New York City

CHAPTER 1

LIVING POSITIVELY

THE BIG LIES

"They" told me that HIV/AIDS was a baffling new disease that was contagious and fatal. "They" said that once someone was exposed to the HIV virus, there was nothing anyone could do—that person would shortly get AIDS and die. Luckily, "they" said, "nice people" didn't have to worry, HIV/AIDS affected only faggots, junkies, whores, and various other "disposable" people.

"They" were wrong. "They" lied. "They" were filled with prejudice. And because of "them," the number of people who are HIV-positive doubles every couple of years—over 20,000,000 at last guess—and *we are now all* living in a world with HIV/AIDS.

The biggest liar in the world is They Say.
—DOUGLAS MALLOCH

TELLING THE TRUTH

Telling the truth about HIV/AIDS isn't easy. It involves talking about very private matters, moral issues, and complex medical and scientific information. We have to talk about sexuality and recreational drug use; the successes and failures of our health-care system; and even deal with our personal views of health, life, death, society, morality, and spirituality.

Certainly these are all controversial subjects that nice society-folk tell us to avoid in polite conversation. I don't wish to be rude or disrespectful of anyone's

For a long time I was ashamed of the way I lived.
—MAE WEST

Did you reform?
—REPORTER

No; I'm just not ashamed anymore.
—MAE WEST

1

sensibilities, but we simply cannot avoid these subjects any longer. Our very lives depend on it.

Some issues that this book brings up might be uncomfortable for you because they involve your religious or moral belief system. That's the whole point. You can believe whatever you want to—this book isn't trying to convert you to any one point of view. Quite the opposite. This book is here to encourage you to take action, and it's vitally important that whatever action you *do take* fits with *your personal belief system*, not with what someone else tells you *should* be right for you.

HIV/AIDS is not a religious or moral issue, it is a public health issue. As such, we have a lot of no-nonsense talking to do to clear up the rumors, dispel the fears, and spread some of the good news about living in a world with HIV/AIDS.

THE GOOD NEWS

Good news about AIDS? How can there be anything good to say about this plague that has caused so much pain and grief for so many wonderful people?

Most stories about HIV/AIDS seem to focus almost exclusively on illness and death. Yet this is not the complete picture. Not by far. HIV/AIDS is increasingly becoming just another treatable, chronic condition.

Finding out that you—or someone you love—is HIV-positive, or has AIDS, is never good news. It starts a chain reaction, and your life will never be the same. But, believe it or not, amazing good can come along as a result of this heartbreak. It can be a wake-up call to live life. As strange as it may seem, for a surprising number of people learning they are HIV-positive leads to a more optimistic and productive life than ever before.

Most of us, most of the time, do not grow because we *want to*, but because we *have to*. It is just

In spite of illness, in spite even of the archenemy sorrow, one can remain alive long past the usual date of disintegration if one is unafraid of change, insatiable in intellectual curiosity, interested in big things, and happy in small ways.

—EDITH WHARTON

too painful and too uncomfortable to keep on doing what we have always done. We can choose to view HIV/AIDS as a painful tragedy, or as a wake-up call to life: an opportunity for some much-needed growth, healing, and change; a driving force for making the most out of life.

Looking back on my own life, I realize that there was a lot that needed changing. Helping my closest friends and family deal with having AIDS or other life-challenging conditions, and being HIV-positive myself, started me on the most difficult—and the most rewarding—period of my life. It forced me to make *major changes* in how I lived. A lot of major changes. Because of these, I now enjoy a better life than I ever dreamed possible.

IS HIV/AIDS FATAL?

Is HIV/AIDS fatal? As strange as it may sound, it all depends on your personal opinion. The term "fatal" means that you will probably die from a thing. But since we are all going to die sometime from something, "fatal" carries with it the idea that it causes death sometime soon. "Soon," however, is a relative term.

If a person was shot in the head, and in a few hours died as a result, then everyone would probably agree that being shot was fatal. If it took, say, a week or even a month to die from these wounds, most people would still agree that this shooting had been fatal.

But what if it had taken five years, or fifty? Even if this person died decades before they otherwise might have, we don't usually think of that original shot, fifty years before, as having been fatal. It just didn't cause the death *soon enough*.

There's a story about the Mummy's Curse that reads "whosoever disturbs this tomb shall die." Eventually anyone who might have disturbed the tomb will die, and then you can blame that death on this curse. A similar story can be told about HIV/AIDS. It might

Again, I am reminded of the words of the Twenty-Sixth Psalm, "Examine me, O Lord, and try me." Disease is surely one of the ways in which we are tried by life and offered the chance to be heroic. Though few of us will win Olympic gold medals or slay dragons, disease can be the spark or gift that allows many of us to live out our personal myths and become heroes.
—BERNIE SIEGEL

take many, many, many years, but eventually everyone with HIV/AIDS will die, and so we can then "prove" that HIV/AIDS was always fatal. The question is, how long does someone have to survive with a "fatal" condition before it isn't considered fatal anymore?

As strange as this may seem, "fatal" is a relative term. It's all about timing. Sean Strub, the founder of *POZ Magazine*, the first national, glossy consumer magazine for people living with HIV/AIDS, put it particularly well:

> If I were a woman and had suffered from breast cancer five years ago, today I would be considered a breast cancer survivor. But even though I have survived HIV for 15 years, I am still considered terminally ill. How much time must pass before I am considered a survivor instead of terminally ill?
>
> Language is important. It influences how society, politicians, and healthcare providers view people with AIDS. Most importantly, it influences how we view ourselves.
>
> If we believe ourselves to be terminally ill, then we void everything else about our lives. Our love, passion, vision, and vitality. Our hopes and dreams. We might as well just plan the funeral and wait to die.
>
> But if we are survivors, we have a future. Something to survive for. Places to go. People to meet. Things to do. Love to share.
>
> There is not a single right answer to any question about AIDS. Ask any group of survivors; each will have as many different successful strategies as there are different individuals.
>
> Every morning I wake up is another morning when I am a survivor. I hope you are too.

A powerful agent is the right word. Whenever we come upon one of those intensely right words the resulting effect is physical as well as spiritual, and electrically prompt.
—MARK TWAIN

HIV/AIDS AS A TREATABLE, CHRONIC CONDITION

Although I don't consider HIV/AIDS to be always fatal, it is still incurable. That doesn't mean it can't be treated effectively. It's important to understand the difference: "Incurable" merely means that doctors and other scientists have not yet discovered a "cure" that removes HIV/AIDS from someone who already has it. Someday they might, but they have not done so yet.

There are many other common treatable, chronic conditions such as diabetes, high blood pressure, arthritis, herpes, and various forms of cancer that are also incurable but treatable. Sometimes these conditions may once again become serious—and could well affect that person's quality and quantity of life—but people have learned to live with them, and continue to enjoy life to the fullest.

For many people with HIV/AIDS, there are a number of treatments that can prevent, cure, or lessen the many symptoms of the diseases that can result from a weakened immune system, and even some treatments that may slow the progress of the HIV virus itself. Every year, more and better treatments are being discovered to prevent and treat the opportunistic infections that challenge those with HIV/AIDS. With each passing year, HIV/AIDS is becoming more and more just another treatable, chronic condition that people can learn to live with. People with HIV/AIDS can, and do, live healthy, productive, fulfilling lives for years, and even decades.

We are not here just to survive and live long . . . We are here to live and know life in its multidimensions, to know life in its richness, in all its variety. And when a man lives multidimensionally, explores all possibilities available, never shrinks back from any challenge, goes, rushes to it, welcomes it, rises to the occasion then life becomes a flame, life blooms.
—BHAGWAN SHREE RAJNEESH

BEATING HIV/AIDS

What does it mean to "beat" HIV/AIDS? Is it living longer than, say, three years after an AIDS diagnosis? Is it never getting sick, or how about becoming HIV-negative?

I like to remind people that *life itself* is a sexually transmitted, progressive, terminal condition. No one gets out of life alive. We are all going to die someday. Even if you read my books, listen to my tapes, and attend my seminars, you are going to die. It could be this week, or next year, or ten years from now, or you could live until you are over a hundred. Whether you are HIV-negative, HIV-positive, or living with AIDS, there is no way of knowing how much longer any one of us will live.

Think about that for a moment. Do you *really* *believe* that you could die this week? Do you *really* *believe* that you could live until you are 110? Try saying out loud "Yes, I could die this week or I could live until I'm a hundred and ten." How did that feel? Did you think that you were telling the truth? You were.

> Do what you can, with what you have, with where you are.
> —THEODORE ROOSEVELT

Even the healthiest and youngest among us only has at best forty thousand days left, absolute tops. Even if they find the miracle cure for HIV/AIDS tomorrow, you are going to die, someday, from some other cause. We all need to take advantage of the remaining good days, months, and years that are left. We all need to learn to *live* while we can.

My own secret to living with HIV/AIDS is quite simple: make the most out of life while you can, do what you can to stay healthy for as long as you can, and when you can't, let go as gracefully as you can, so you make things as pleasant as possible for those left behind.

> Healing is possible, even when a cure is not.
> —BILL MOYERS

"Healing" is more than fixing one, small broken part of a person's body or killing off one small virus; it is about helping a person to become a more complete human being. Healing does not mean being "cured" from all your symptoms and living forever. As Fran Peavey wrote in her book, *A Shallow Pool of Time*:

> The victory is in how you handled whatever came along, not just winning the length-of-life battle. Victory could well be getting through this in a friendly and

gracious way, letting people love you, staying real through whatever came. In other words, refusing to give in to pretense or bullshit. To me, that is the victory in every day—including your last one.

WE ALL RESPOND A LITTLE DIFFERENTLY

Each person who has ever lived is a little different from everyone else. Part of this is genetic, part of this is what we have been exposed to. Even identical twins rapidly develop measurably different immune systems because of the subtle differences in how they have been exposed to different things.

Without deviation, progress is not possible.
—FRANK ZAPPA

Each person responds just a little bit differently to each specific disease or environmental condition. This is the way that evolution works. There is supposed to be enough variation or "genetic diversity" so that given almost any change in the environment, at least *some people*, somewhere, will be able to survive and reproduce the species. It's ironic that Adolph Hitler's idea of "racial purity" could have limited humankind to such a narrow spectrum of diversity that everyone could have been wiped out by one really bad flu season.

Throughout all of history, for all diseases, there have been some people who have been very susceptible to each particular disease. Once infected with the smallest amount, these unfortunate folks get sick and die quickly. At the other end of the spectrum, there have always been at least a few folks who, for some reason or another, seem to be almost immune to each particular disease, and can be exposed again and again, never getting sick. Of course, most everyone else lies somewhere in the middle, where they are to some degree more resistant or more susceptible.

It is reasonable to assume the same will be true for HIV/AIDS. We know there are some people who get infected with a small amount of HIV one time, and quickly become HIV-positive, get sick, and die. At the other end of the spectrum, there is a group of prostitutes in Uganda who have somehow remained HIV-negative, even though they have had unsafe sex many times each day for years with people who are known to be HIV-positive or to have AIDS.

In between these two extremes, there are many people who test HIV-positive for years or even decades without getting serious symptoms. Even those who do develop "full-blown AIDS" have been known to live for over a decade.

A study from the San Francisco Department of Health of 562 gay men with well-documented dates of becoming HIV-positive shows that after 12½ years, almost one-third had not progressed to having AIDS. A statistical model from Johns Hopkins University is even more encouraging. It indicates that some HIV-positive people are likely to stay healthy for 20 years or longer.

THE "RIGHT CHOICE"

Religions are different roads converging upon the same point. What does it matter that we take different roads so long as we reach the same goal?
—MAHATMA GANDHI

For some reason, most of us like to believe in the myth of the simple black-and-white answer. Either something is true, or it isn't; something either works, or it doesn't. Most of the important things in life just don't work that way. Each of us must find for ourselves whom to fall in love with, what to do for a living, how to fit in with the universe, what sort of life-style to lead.

What is the "right" way to live with HIV/AIDS? Again, just like living without HIV/AIDS, there are no wrong answers, but there do tend to be more questions that have to be faced sooner than perhaps others need to face them.

Which choices along the path are right for you? The answer to all these questions is that there isn't a single answer. I hope that this book will help each of you find your own path toward a fuller, richer, and more healthy life.

Each person is unique and we must all find what is best for ourselves. Just as in the rest of life, there are no short and snappy miracle answers that are right for everyone. It depends on who you are, what's important to you, what you believe in, what your needs are, and a thousand other factors.

Not only is there no single right answer; there are no wrong answers either. I have found that there are as many different ways of living with HIV/AIDS as there are those of us who must do so. Everybody may choose what's right for him or her at that moment. An example: for some following a vegetarian diet is both healthy and enjoyable; for others, it is neither.

No matter how much you love someone, you cannot force them to cope with HIV/AIDS the way that you want them to. As heartbreaking as it may be at times, you cannot force an alcoholic to stop drinking, a fat person to lose weight, or a nonbeliever to follow a religious or spiritual path. All one can do is to use the quiet power of example.

The absence of alternatives clears the mind marvelously.
—HENRY KISSINGER

LIFE IS SERVED "BUFFET STYLE"

Auntie Mame said that "Life is a banquet, and most poor sons-of-bitches are starving." I like to think this means life is served "buffet style," and you get to take from it what you want from today's selections, as you want it, and leave behind the stuff you don't like.

Most books about living with HIV/AIDS take some "position." They say that AZT is either good or bad for you; or that a macrobiotic diet is either the right or wrong way to go; or that you should do one thing and should not do something else.

I cannot recommend any wonder drugs or magical treatments. I do not offer recipes for tofu milk shakes or New Age mantras. But just like beating

It is common sense to take a method and try it. If it fails, admit it frankly and try another. But above all, try something.
—FRANKLIN D. ROOSEVELT

cancer, or a heart attack, or a stroke, or almost anything else, statistically, the most important factors are non-medical ones, such as changing your attitudes and life-style. There are many things that can be done, in addition to whatever medical treatments you may choose, to improve the quality and quantity of your life.

The purpose of this book is to help you, the reader, take a look at these things, offer up some alternatives that perhaps you might not have encountered or considered before, and help you in the process of figuring out what's right for you.

BEING HEALTHY

Finding the right medical treatments is a vital but very incomplete part of the action one can take to cope with HIV disease. It is tremendously important that we do whatever we can to keep our body, mind, emotions, and spirit working as well as possible. We must focus on taking many small actions that add up to improving both the quality and quantity of our lives, and avoiding those actions that do not.

The body, mind, emotions, and spirit are linked together. What we call the "immune system" is really an incredibly complex interrelated system affected by countless hormones and other chemical triggers released by the brain, central nervous system, and the rest of the body. Being peaceful or angry releases dramatically different sets of hormones, each of which will have a profoundly distinct chemical effect on every aspect of one's body.

People talk about "being worried sick" or losing the "will to live" and dying after some serious setback. Whether you call it "Type-A behavior," "psychosomatic illness," or "a broken heart," a person's emotional attitudes and beliefs definitely can cause disease and even death.

And more importantly for us, a person's emotional attitudes and beliefs can help cure disease and work miracles. Who hasn't heard of stories like the one about the petite mother who, with adrenaline pumping, could lift a car off the ground to free her little baby?

What I am describing is far more than the mere "wishful thinking" or the "faith healing" reported in the supermarket tabloids and on "evangelical" TV scams. Countless scientific studies have shown that changing one's attitudes and life-style are the most important factors in recovering from all major illnesses—from cancer to heart attacks, from strokes to drug addiction, to practically everything else.

I'm a big fan of finding people who have achieved what I want (health, happiness, longevity) and trying to copy what they are doing right. Surely one of the best indicators of "being healthy" is living for a long time, so let's look at some groups of people who are doing just that.

First, let's look at some remarkable HIV-negative people who must be doing something right: In a five-year study of 96 healthy, independent "centenarians," or people who are more than 100 years old, Professors Leonard Poon and Gloria Clayton from Georgia commented in 1992 that "you might think that the common thread would be something like diet or exercise or genetics, but these were not among the four main traits that . . . [caused longevity. The common factors were] optimism, engagement or commitment to something that they're interested in, activity or mobility, and the ability to adapt to loss."

Another recent study of HIV-negative people with heart disease, reported in the *New England Journal of Medicine*, showed that the greatest factor in surviving was how strongly the patient measured on objective psychological tests measuring optimism and sense of humor.

Only in the last few years has the HIV/AIDS com-

You see things; and you say, "Why?" But I dream things that never were; and I say, "Why not?"
—GEORGE BERNARD SHAW

munity turned serious attention to studying a large number of people living with HIV/AIDS who were doing well, to see what they were doing right. My personal opinion is that this is the single most important area for study—more so than any pharmaceutical drug trial—in the care and treatment of people with HIV/AIDS.

At the 1992 international HIV/AIDS conference in Amsterdam we heard the first of these reports. A study of people who had survived with AIDS for more than ten years showed that the most important factors influencing good health are people's general attitude and life-style rather than the specific treatments that they followed.

WE CAN LOOK TO OUR HEROES

Like all disasters throughout history—from fires, floods, and famines, to earthquakes, hurricanes, and wars—there have been wonderful stories of ordinary people rising to the occasion and doing extraordinary things. There are stories of age-old wounds being healed, and of fractured families and communities being brought together.

It was all done by Christ and Gandhi and St. Francis of Assisi and Dr. King. They did it all. We don't have to think about new ideas; we just have to implement what they said, just get the work done.
—CESAR CHAVEZ

Along my own journey in learning to live in a world with HIV/AIDS, I have been fortunate to meet and work with some truly remarkable people who learned through trial and error how to beat the system, stay healthy, and improve the quality of their lives. It's my hope to pass along to you some of what they have taught me.

The credit for the wisdom in this book belongs to them. I am more like a reporter—the pragmatic observer reporting what has worked for a very large number of people living with HIV/AIDS. What's more, none of the ideas in this book are really new at all. If they were, they wouldn't be nearly as valuable as those that are proven, tried, and true.

These are our love stories. They are the legacy

of AIDS. They must be told and retold, so that the lessons that these courageous people learned at such a great cost will not go to waste. They have blazed a trail for us so that we can go on to make our entire world a better place to live.

What doesn't kill me makes me stronger.
—NIETZSCHE

CHAPTER 2

THE EIGHT KEY POINTS OF LIVING POSITIVELY

BEGINNING ACTION

Rule Number One is: don't sweat the small stuff. Rule Number Two is: it's all small stuff. And if you can't fight and you can't flee, go with the flow.
—R.S. ELIOT

Never put off till tomorrow what you can do the day after tomorrow.
—MARK TWAIN

Learning how to live with HIV/AIDS is not easy. In fact, it's probably the most difficult thing that you will ever have to cope with. There are just so many facts to learn and even more really tough decisions to make. Luckily, you don't have to do everything all at once.

Things may seem really urgent, but almost anything can wait *a little bit* until you get some more information and skills. You don't have to figure out what treatments to follow *today*, or how you're going to pay for this expensive new "hobby" of having HIV/AIDS, or how to handle all those difficult emotional and social issues that invariably come up. This doesn't mean you can put things off indefinitely; it just means you can take the time you need to work through this book.

You will notice that I didn't say "read this book." This book is about giving you information and skills to use, not just to understand. It's easy to be overwhelmed and get stuck. The secret to getting unstuck is committing to action. Both physical action and mental action. Get out of bed. Get out of your home. Read just one page. Try just one suggested activity. Don't overdo it, but even a little progress feels a lot better than being stuck.

Forward movement builds up and keeps us going. My father was a professor of the history of science at Yale University. I learned early on about Sir Isaac Newton's second law: "An object at rest will remain at rest and an object in motion will remain in motion unless acted upon by an outside force." This applies just as much to people as it does to protons.

W. H. Murray, the great explorer, was once asked to what he attributed the success of his group, the Scottish Himalayan Expedition, in climbing to the top of Mount Everest. Murray replied:

> Until one is committed, there is hesitancy, the chance to draw back, always ineffectiveness. Concerning all acts of initiative (and creation) there is one elementary truth, the ignorance of which kills countless ideas and splendid plans: that the moment one definitely commits oneself, then Providence moves too. All sorts of things occur to help one that would never otherwise have occurred. A whole stream of events issues from the decision, raising in one's favor all manner of unforeseen incidents, and meetings and material assistance, which no man could have dreamed would have come his way. I have learned a deep respect for one of Goethe's couplets:

> "Whatever you can do
> or dream you can, begin it.
> Boldness has genius,
> Power and magic in it."

THE "RIGHT" ANSWERS

There is no one "right" answer that works for everyone, all the time. Each person must find what's right for himself.

This phrase is repeated over and over again, in one form or another, in every section of this book. Over the years, countless people have asked me about some new research or drug or treatment or diet or

The most important thing is—don't just read this book, use it. Do some things. Try them out. Find out if they work for you, if they produce uplifting results. If so, do some more. If not, throw it away [and try something else].

—PETER McWILLIAMS

A step in the wrong direction is better than staying on the spot all your life. Once you're moving forward you can correct your course as you go. Your automatic guidance system cannot guide you when you're standing still.

—MAXWELL MALTZ

book or guru, hoping to find the magic answer. And again, I repeat to them this phrase: *There is no one "right" answer* . . .

I'm a very practical, pragmatic guy. I look at the people who seem to be successful in living with HIV/AIDS, and I try to find out what they might be doing right. Perhaps whatever it is that they are doing might work for me, too. I also try to look at people who maybe aren't doing so well, and try to see what things they might be doing that aren't working so well for them. Perhaps these are things that I, too, am doing that I might want to avoid as well.

The problem is, most people have no idea *what it is* that is working so well for them. Even worse, many of the most outspoken people are absolutely sure that one particular thing that they are doing is the "right" magic answer, and that everyone else should be doing this thing as well.

Although there might not be any magic answers, there do seem to be some key questions and issues that a lot of these folks who are successful at living with HIV/AIDS seem to be addressing. I've grouped these together into eight key points, or areas, and expanded on each one of these in the remaining eight chapters of this book.

THE EIGHT KEY POINTS OF LIVING POSITIVELY

1. Regardless of what might have happened in the past, or could possibly happen in the future, you are alive right now. Focusing on living in the present moment, while building the best future you can, is the most powerful thing anyone can ever do.

   Only the present is real. The past no longer exists and the future hasn't happened yet. Although the issues that come up may be substantial, the fears behind them are not. Regardless of what we might call our unpleasant feelings, they all boil down to some form of fear. Like shadows, all fears will disappear when examined under the light of how things really are right now.

2. Even the healthiest people do not get very long on this planet, so you might as well make the most of it and enjoy your stay. Don't take things too seriously; have fun, laugh, and make a conscious effort to enjoy every day to the fullest. Take the time to savor the journey, not just the accomplishments.

   Choose to focus on the positive good news in life and on the love in everybody, including yourself. Don't dwell too much on the occasional difficulties and fears. Seeing the glass as half-full, rather than half-empty, creates more happiness and peace for you and those around you.

3. HIV/AIDS can be too tough and confusing to deal with alone. Luckily, you don't have to. You may be surprised how supportive friends, family, coworkers, and the rest of your community can be in helping you deal with all the everyday difficulties, errands, annoyances, contradictions, and fears.

   Regardless of how bad (or good) things might be for you, helping someone who's having a hard time—even if it's only reaching out to them with a phone call— will help you forget your own troubles and make you grateful for your good fortune. It also makes you both feel better. Remember how good it feels to help others, and give someone else that opportunity too, by sometimes letting others help you.

4. Do things that are healthy for your body, mind, and spirit, and avoid those that are not. Being healthy is about balance, variety, and moderation in all the aspects of your life. Learn to listen to your body; it may be trying to tell you something. Avoid focusing too much attention on any one small piece—you might be ignoring the larger whole.

5. "Knowledge is Power." In an ideal world, your doctor and the rest of your health-care team would devote all their skills and energy to you. But try as they might, they have hundreds (or even thousands) of other patients and other conditions to keep up with. You have a much smaller caseload, and you can—if you really do your homework—know more about your personal condition than any doctor or other expert could.

6. Take an active role in your health care. Letting even the best health-care professional choose your treatment is like letting a travel agent choose where you're going on vacation. Both can have invaluable input, knowledge, and experience, but they can't know what's right for you unless you ask questions, do your homework, learn all you can, evaluate your options, and communicate how you feel.

Sometimes these folks forget that their main job is to advise you, coach you, and provide you with the information you need to make your own choices and take your own actions. "Reeducate" those who want to dictate "what you have to do." You don't have to do anything. There are no magic answers in life that are right for all people at all times.

Seek out people who will listen to you, respect you, and work with you as a member of your team. Work in collaboration with them, but don't let them bully you into doing anything that you really don't believe in. Remember that it is your body; you make the final decisions; you have the right to keep asking "why?" and the right to say "no" to anything that you don't fully understand and agree with.

7. Reduce stress and find daily activities that give you some inner peace and quiet time. Each of us finds serenity in a different way, and only you can know what's right for you. Some people find it through exercise, yoga, or meditation. Others find it by doing something artistic, creative, or by communing with nature. Many enjoy some form of spiritual, religious, or philosophical path.

8. Life is a process of growth and change. Along the way, each of us has developed our own unique "survival kit" to cope with whatever stuff we needed to. We carry with us the scars and baggage from this process. It's important not only to pick up new experiences, ideas, possessions, friends, and new ways of looking at things, but also to edit out the old ones that no longer work for us.

This "spring cleaning" process of simplifying life and reevaluating goals, priorities, and beliefs is seldom easy—particularly when the issues are family, finances, career, material possessions, life's purpose, and even our own mortality—but it can be incredibly rewarding and liberating.

CHAPTER 3

LIVING IN THE PRESENT MOMENT

> **1.** Regardless of what might have happened in the past, or could possibly happen in the future, you are alive right now. Focusing on living in the present moment, while building the best future you can, is the most powerful thing anyone can ever do.
>
> Only the present is real. The past no longer exists and the future hasn't happened yet. Although the issues that come up may be substantial, the fears behind them are not. Regardless of what we might call our unpleasant feelings, they all boil down to some form of fear. Like shadows, all fears will disappear when examined under the light of how things really are right now.

FEAR: THE MOST CONTAGIOUS, DEADLY DISEASE

The fear of HIV/AIDS is far worse than any of the actual medical conditions that the HIV virus can cause. Many people who are HIV-negative, HIV-positive, or living with AIDS live in terror because they believe some of the sensationalized half-truths reported in the mass media. As hard as many responsible people might try sometimes, anything really important about HIV/AIDS is far too complex to be able to be reported in the short "sound bite" or "information graphic" formats that are so popular today.

Fear is probably the most contagious and deadly

Considering how dangerous everything is, nothing is really very frightening.
—GERTRUDE STEIN
Everybody's Autobiography

of all human conditions. It can be spread worldwide
instantly through the miracle of modern communications. It can cause hatred and violence, and, worst of
all, the fear itself slowly chokes the life force out of
us.

Living with HIV/AIDS can be pretty scary stuff,
but then again, so can life. On one level at least, everything is not necessarily *just fine*. There are so many
choices to make, so many things that need to be done,
and even more things that we need to stop doing.
Sometimes it seems that everything has to be done
right away.

We might have physical aches and pains, or a
slew of day-to-day difficulties dealing with our friends,
family, finances, health-care professionals, and the various bureaucracies. There are medical choices on what
sort of treatments to follow, there are life-style choices
on how to live, there are practical matters of how to
pay for treatments, and there is a whole life of unfinished business that now seems even more pressing.

We have to deal with all the tough issues and
difficulties that everyone else has to deal with *eventually*, if they live long enough. In our case, however,
we were promoted to life's accelerated, advanced class,
so we get to face these issues that much sooner and
more intensely than most.

THE MORE YOU RESIST,
THE MORE IT PERSISTS

It's one of those unfailing rules of nature: the more
you resist focusing on something, the more it persists
in drawing your attention. It's just like the children's
story about a magic spell that will give anyone unlimited wealth and power. The only catch was, if you
were to think about a purple elephant, you had to wait
an hour before you could use this magic spell.

Whenever we try to *not think* about something,
that's just what we keep focusing on. Our minds can

be filled with lots of *purple elephants*: that person we *never, ever* want to see or speak to again, our latest test results, all sorts of visions of illness and death, that pile of unpaid bills, nameless fears and emotions of all kinds, and even those unhealthy (but sometimes fun) things we used to do.

All of these things can rent a lot of space in our heads. The best way to exorcise these demons is to confront them. Bertrand Russell, the English mathematician, logician, and philosopher, who was roughly a peer to Albert Einstein, offered this nugget of sound advice in his book *The Conquest of Happiness*:

> When some misfortune threatens, consider seriously and deliberately what is the very worst that could possibly happen. Having looked this possible misfortune in the face, give yourself sound reasons for thinking that after all it would be no such terrible disaster. Such reasons always exist, since at the worst nothing that happens to oneself has any cosmic importance. When you have looked for some time steadily at the worst possibility and have said to yourself with real conviction, "Well, after all, that would not matter so very much," you will find that your worry diminishes to a quite extraordinary extent. It may be necessary to repeat the process a few times, but in the end, if you have shirked nothing in facing the worst possible issue, you will find that your worry disappears altogether and is replaced by a kind of exhilaration.

Years ago, I told myself not to worry about a devil. I remember thinking that there's no force of evil out stalking the planet. That, I told myself, is all in my mind. Then I realized this is not good news. Since every thought creates experience, there's no worse place it could possibly be.
—MARIANNE WILLIAMSON
A Return to Love

In Hollywood they understand how fears work: Hollywood movie monsters always lurk in the foggy shadows. Half-unseen, they can terrify our imagination. If these monsters were brought out clearly into the light of day, we could begin to understand them. Our fears would evaporate, and we could learn to live with *whatever* beasts were out there.

ONE DAY AT A TIME

*And the only
measure of your
words and your
deeds, will be the
love you leave
behind, when you're
gone.*

—FRED SMALL
"Everything
Possible"

When I was four or five, my mother taught me to swim. Eventually, the time came for me to let go of the safety near the edge of the pool and swim the few feet to my mom. I knew I could do that. I swam and swam, but my mom kept seeming to be just a few inches farther away, so I kept swimming. When I finally reached her, she gave me a big hug, and I saw that I had swum the entire length of that small pool— she had been running backward just as fast as I had been swimming forward. I would never have dared to try and swim so far, but I knew I could swim just a few more strokes.

In twelve-step fellowships like Alcoholics Anonymous, they talk about living "one day at a time." At first, I thought they were playing the same kind of trick: If you don't think you can stop drinking for the rest of your life, how about *not drinking today*, or until after lunch, and then eventually the days would add up to decades.

*Do what you are
doing.*

—CICERO

There is a lot more to "one day at a time" than this. It's about seizing each day—*carpe diem*, as they say in Latin—and focusing on the present moment. It's about being conscious of everything you are doing. It's about noticing the details, the textures, the lighting, the smells, the flavors of life, and not just breezing through on autopilot.

TIME

Whether you are HIV-negative, HIV-positive, or living with AIDS, *time* is our most limited resource.

Time is very democratic. Every person gets exactly twenty-four hours in each day. Everyone from the very richest to the poorest gets exactly 86,400 seconds to use each day. After taking out a rather large chunk for sleeping, we are left with only having something like 60,000 seconds each day to live our lives with.

The human body is remarkable, it can do *thousands* of things at the same time. It not only controls all the muscles and internal functions, it also processes all the sights, sounds, smells, tastes, and feelings even better than today's fastest supercomputers.

Unfortunately, the human brain isn't very good at working on more than one primary thing at a time. Sure, most of us can chew gum while we walk down the street. But when it comes to bigger tasks that require our conscious attention, we are pretty much limited to one task at a time.

Thinking—meaning what we choose to focus our conscious mind on—is, unfortunately, one of these one-at-a-time tasks. If you choose to spend any given second thinking about the past or about the future, then you aren't able to spend that second living in the present.

Of course, we all have to plan for the future *to some extent*, and we all want both to learn from the past and enjoy our happy memories. But actions only happen in those seconds left over. Dwelling too much on the past or future is a form of death in and of itself. Living in the present means that your efforts need to be focused on your actions today.

BACK TO THE PRESENT

One of my teachers in helping me learn to live with HIV/AIDS had a very annoying habit. She would interrupt me—right in the middle of my complaining—to innocently ask me what time it was. I would check my watch and answer her, almost without thinking, and go right on with my complaints. Then she would ask me what day it was. Again, I would check my watch—just to make sure—and I would answer her.

Then I would realize that she had, once again, tricked me. She would continue by asking, "What are you doing right now?" Eventually, I would get the hint

First I was dying to finish high school and start college.

And then I was dying to finish college and start working.

And then I was dying to marry and have children.

And then I was dying for my children to grow old enough for school so I could return to work.

And then I was dying to retire.

And now, I am dying . . .

And suddenly I realize I forgot to live.

—ANONYMOUS

that she meant that I needed to return my focus to the present moment, not the fearful future or guilty past.

As a little kid, one of the very few blasphemies that I would be scolded for, was saying that I *couldn't wait* until some special day in the future, or, say, that I *wished it was next Friday already*. I would be told in no uncertain terms that we didn't get very long on this planet, and that we ought to make the most of each moment, and not waste any of it.

What day is it today? What time is it? Where are you? What are you doing right now? The answers to these questions may seem simplistic, but they are vital. *Probably the most important single key to living positively is living in the present moment.* Yesterday is only a memory and tomorrow is only a dream. Today is real. All fears and worries live in the future, things that only might happen sometime later . . . or then again, they might not. But if you let them, these fears will rob you of the only time that you really have— right now.

TAKING ACTION, NOT JUST GAINING UNDERSTANDING

So far, in this book, there has been a lot of reading, concepts, and philosophy, and not a lot of action. Unfortunately, one only gets so much benefit from *understanding* how to live with HIV/AIDS. The real payoff comes from *taking action*. As important as laying the groundwork has been, it is now time to stop *reading* for a bit, and start *doing*.

If you're like me, it can be pretty tempting just to keep on reading, and promise to come back to action points sometime later. Don't wait too long. That would be like going to the gym and *watching* the aerobics class week after week so that you could *understand* what to do. This doesn't help very much. The only benefits come from *doing things*. Even doing *just a little*, or doing it *badly* is much better than *under-*

standing it perfectly, but not taking action.

My goal is to give you the motivation, tools, and the skills to live with HIV/AIDS and find your own answers. Just like everything else in this book, there is no one way of doing things. Not every exercise will be appropriate or important for each reader, but it's often tough to tell which areas hold the most benefit until you've tried them.

To begin, you will need a place to record your thoughts and make various lists. I am a writer, so I like to write things down in a notebook or on my Macintosh PowerBook computer. Maybe for you, talking into an inexpensive tape recorder works better, or perhaps working with someone who will help you put things down on paper.

Buying some form of notebook with blank lined pages is certainly the easiest and least expensive option. I suggest one of those 200-page bound composition books that only cost a couple of bucks. In some ways I'm not very rigidly organized myself, so I date each entry, write down as much as possible, tape or staple business cards and scraps of paper in, and never tear pages out. That way, I have only *one place* to look when I need to find what some doctor said to me, or the phone number for some program. It also acts as a kind of *diary* that I can look back on to see what I was thinking and how far I've come.

Whatever method you choose, the important thing is that you start *using something* to help you organize your thoughts, questions, concerns, and things to do. You will want to have some record of what you did so that you can refer back to it in the future.

This will be "your HIV notebook":

Give a man a fish, and he will eat for a day.
Teach a man to fish, and he will eat for a lifetime.
—TAOIST PROVERB

I always say, keep a diary and someday it'll keep you.
—MAE WEST

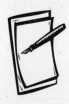

Remember, your HIV notebook is solely for *your benefit.* You need to be able to write things down without worrying how other people will feel about them. This isn't English class. Spelling and neatness *do not* count. Nothing has to be too long or fancy, or even in complete sentences. The only requirement is that you be able to understand it when you refer back to it in the future.

The hardest part is starting. So let's just jump in and begin. Take a quiet, tranquil moment for yourself. Take a deep breath, focus and center your thoughts, and begin . . .

Begin difficult things while they are easy. Do great things when they are small. The difficult things of the world must once have been easy; the great things must once have been small . . . A thousand mile journey begins with one step.

—LAO-TZU

 How are you right now? Focusing on the present, look at your body, mind, and spirit. What are you particularly happy with, and what areas are going right? Make a list of at least twenty things that you are excited about or grateful for. Do it now.

LEARNING FROM THE PAST

Those who cannot remember the past are condemned to repeat it.

—GEORGE SANTAYANA

One of the few smart ideas to come out of war is the "after action review" where after each battle—or as they euphemistically call them "military action"—the various generals and decision-makers review what happened to see what they did right, what they might have done differently, and what they could learn from the experience. The purpose is not to rehash the past or to place blame, but to learn from the past so that they might be even better next time.

Apple Computer, one of the most successful American companies of the last decade, used to ask a trick question during employment interviews: "What are the three biggest mistakes that you have made over the last ten years?" The rationale was that if you hadn't made any really big mistakes, then it was a *very bad sign.* Either you were taking things too safely, and would not risk trying to grow or make things better, or you didn't notice or admit to these inevitable mistakes, which was even worse, because then you couldn't learn from them.

What are some of the biggest mistakes that you have made, and what did you learn from them? Is it possible that if you hadn't made these "mistakes," you might not be as good a person as you are today?

For me, the "after action review" is a particularly valuable tool, because sometimes I forget things, and I really hate to make the same mistakes twice. Once, shame on them; twice, shame on me.

Before I go to bed, I like to review my day, and see what I did right and what I might do differently next time. This process really helps me feel good about myself, regardless of the day's outcome.

In the last twenty-four hours, what ten or more things, no matter how minor, did you do that were right in some way? Things that help make you or the world just a little bit better or healthier? Things that you can be proud of? Don't forget to give yourself credit on this list for writing this list.

UNFINISHED BUSINESS

There is nothing that can ever be done to change what actually happened in the past. We can, however, choose to change the way we think about things that happened in the past.

Instead of focusing on the guilt and resentments, we can choose to look at the long-term benefits of "this wonderful opportunity for growth and change." Perhaps we couldn't have become the sort of people we are today if we hadn't had the opportunity to go through these experiences.

Always forgive your enemies—nothing annoys them so much.
—OSCAR WILDE

If someone did something unforgivable to us many years ago, we can choose to carry with us anger and resentment toward them, and maybe even worry ourselves literally sick or try to "get even" with them.

Alternatively, we could decide to give them our very own version of a presidential pardon on humanitarian grounds—not to make it easier *for them*, but to make it *easier for us*. That way we don't have to carry around all that anger inside of ourselves. Regardless of what they did, by now our anger and resentment certainly does *us* more harm than it does them.

It might not "be fair" that they should get off scot-free, but whether you call it God, Karma, Tao, or the balance of the universe, things have an uncanny way of catching up with people. What goes around, comes around.

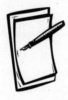 *Make a list of people, either living or dead, that if you were to see them in a supermarket, you would either change aisles to avoid them, or secretly hope that a gallon of chocolate syrup would pour all over them, or worse. Be prepared to add to this list over time. This is a list of people from your past that you have some unfinished business with.*

GETTING THINGS DONE

Life is like playing a violin in public and learning the instrument as one goes on.
—SAMUEL BUTLER

Living with HIV/AIDS can be a full-time job. In fact, at times it seems that it would be nice to have a full-time staff to help deal with all the phone calls, appointments, correspondence, paperwork, accounting, and research that needs to get done. I would love to be waited on like some old-style Hollywood Diva, and devote all my energy and skill to my most important project: being healthy and living life.

Realistically though, HIV/AIDS is expensive, even without this grandiose stuff. But all those chores still have to get done. And like it or not, you're the one responsible for doing them. Others may *help*, but sometimes even your nearest and closest friends won't be able to come through for you all the time.

For some reason, it seems harder to solve your own problems than it does someone else's, mainly because it is harder to get a perspective. Try taking a step back, and think of yourself helping your *very best friend*. For now, we're not going to worry about actually doing any of these things or solving any of these problems. We just want to know what they are.

 Your best friend asked you: "I have unlimited time, please give me a complete list of all the things that I can do to help and problems to help you solve." Make two "laundry lists," one of specific "to do" items and the other of larger issues or problems to be dealt with.

Living with HIV/AIDS does seem to generate quite a long list of things to work on, doesn't it? Remember, the purpose of this list isn't to beat yourself up for not having done them all yet, nor should you try to do them all right away. In fact, maybe there are some things on this list that aren't worth doing at all.

There are three factors that affect when—or if—you should work on each of these items:

1. How important is the benefit *to you* if this thing gets accomplished?
2. What are the urgency, availability, or other time considerations involved?
3. How much energy, time, money, or other resources will it require?

One reason we often don't get around to things is because, quite frankly, they just aren't important to us. Perhaps we feel they *should* be important to us, or they are important to someone else, but pleasing these other people just isn't worth doing the task. In that case, scratch it off the list. Life is too short to waste any of it doing unimportant things, and you've decided that *this* simply isn't important enough to you.

The longer I live, the more importance I attach to a man's ability to manage and discipline himself . . . The man with the capacity for self-discipline can tell himself to do the truly important things first. Therefore, if there is not enough time to go around and something must be neglected, it will be the less essential task.

*—RAY KROC
founder of
McDonald's*

I think most people, when they get to the end of their lives, don't look back and wish that they had spent *more time* at the office or more time watching TV. The important thing is to remember this while we are alive and can schedule time for doing the really important things and spending time with the people we love.

Another reason we don't get around to really important things is that a lot of unimportant things get done first. Since you can't do *everything* in life, perhaps you need to cut out some less-important things that creep into your schedule because they have urgent time requirements.

Now, using these three concepts, go back over your "to do" list and scratch out everything that you can. For those important but not time-urgent items, set your own deadlines, for example, "by next Friday, set up appointment with the AIDS project to review insurance."

Now that you have a much more manageable list, you might want to recopy it so you can refer to it more easily and note those items that are particularly important, urgent, or easy to do. Do them first.

Lastly, there's the problem of resources. Often projects will take so much time or cost so much money that we put off starting until we have enough of both to complete the project. One solution is to break each of these down into smaller, bite-sized chunks that can be tackled. For example, filing your taxes is too much to do in one sitting, so you might break down the task into smaller tasks—like getting the correct forms, reading the instructions, finding all the medical bills or the bank statements, etc.

Sometimes the problem isn't that the task is too big, but we just don't know how to solve it. A useful problem-solving technique in this case is to write down (in your notebook, of course) a list of all options and include even the most extreme, even if they are not possible or not acceptable. Even the wackiest ideas might help you think of something else that just might work, or at least help you put the problem in perspective.

Remember, you don't actually have to do anything about this until sometime later. If some other issue comes up, write it down.

For example, let's say you were not able to pay your phone bill; some of the options you might write down could be:

I am a great believer in luck, and I find the harder I work the more I have of it.

—*STEPHEN LEACOCK*

- Borrow from someone
- Steal from somewhere
- Sell something
- Earn it somehow
- Talk honestly with the phone company
- Lie to the phone company
- Do nothing
- Give up/resign/run away/hide/move/escape
- Kill myself/attack "them"

Imagine what some hypothetical, average, prudent, "normal" person who was in this identical situation and had the same information would do? Imagine what somebody who is really smart and wise, such as Einstein, Gandhi, Jesus, a wise grandmother, or someone you admire would suggest?

CONFRONTING THE BIGGEST DEMONS

Now that we have rooted ourselves firmly in the present, learned a little from our past mistakes, and given ourselves credit for what we are doing right today, it is time to confront some of those fearful demons that we mentioned a few pages ago.

The only thing we have to fear is fear itself.

—*FRANKLIN D. ROOSEVELT*

Hopefully the list is much shorter now that you've worked through this chapter. Many of our unnamed fears have been converted into very doable items to work on. Nevertheless, all of us have some bigger fears. Let's take a look.

Face the thing you fear, and you do away with that fear.
—RALPH WALDO EMERSON

What are you afraid of? What worries draw you out of the present into a fearful future? Don't worry about being macabre or grim. Include those that "maybe" should be on your list "a little." Leave room for a long list. Here are some fears you might want to take a look at:

- Getting sick; being in pain; suffering with a long illness

- Losing your looks; being unsightly; looking old

- Being an outcast; stigmatized; rejected; abandoned; alone; the last apple on the tree

- Having no one to take care of you

- Running out of money and/or insurance benefits

- Losing your mind

- Losing your sight or your mobility

- Not being self-sufficient; being vulnerable; losing autonomy and self-control; losing your dignity and privacy; being unable to take care of yourself; being a burden on those you love

- Not having done enough; not being good enough; not handling things well enough

- Leaving unfinished business; not having made a difference with your life; not leaving a good enough legacy; being forgotten;

not having the time/energy to accomplish all that you had hoped for

- Not having had children or not being there to see them grow up

- Not being able to take care of your kids/ your business/your project/your pet/your (fill in the blank). What will become of them when you're not there to take care of them?

- Fear of death; of dying; and of what happens after death

Getting to the bottom of this list can be pretty tough. I think most of us will find that we're afraid of a lot more things than we thought we were. But remember, these fears are not facts; they are not real. These things have not happened, and most of them never will. Now go through this list again, and stare down each monster, one by one.

What is the very worst that could possibly happen? Even if this were to happen, is it possible that things would be OK, at least on some larger level?

Plan for the worst Hope for the best And aim down the middle
—*ANONYMOUS*

Now that we've faced the worst possibilities, it's time to focus on the brighter side.

CHAPTER 4

ENJOYING THE JOURNEY AND FOCUSING ON THE POSITIVE

2 Even the healthiest people do not get very long on this planet, so you might as well make the most of it and enjoy your stay. Don't take things too seriously; have fun, laugh, and make a conscious effort to enjoy every day to the fullest. Take the time to savor the journey, not just the accomplishments.

Choose to focus on the positive good news in life and on the love in everybody, including yourself. Don't dwell too much on the occasional difficulties and fears. Seeing the glass as half-full, rather than half-empty, creates more happiness and peace for you and those around you.

Each player must accept the cards life deals him or her. But once they are in hand, he or she alone must decide how to play the cards in order to win the game.

—VOLTAIRE

One of my goals in life is to become a "centenarian," someone who is over 100 years old. I like to think my chances are pretty good. Last year, I passed the one-third mark with a big party to celebrate 33 years and 4 months! After all, the next big milestone is the halfway point, and that won't be until 2010.

In America today, over 12% of the population is already over 65 years old, and the average life expectancy is over 75 years. Worldwide, there are more than 40,000 people alive today who have exceeded my goal, many by quite a bit. According to *The Guinness Book of Records*, Shigechiyo Izumi lived until he was well over 120 years.

I will admit, none of these folks have been living

with HIV/AIDS since they were twenty-something, but they had to survive lots of other deadly plagues in their time.

But even Shigechiyo Izumi only got a total of 43,832 days to make the most of, and we almost certainly have *a lot fewer*. Older people, like their younger counterparts who are dealing with life-challenging conditions, often have a better perspective than most. A wonderful 81-year-old woman from Louisville, Kentucky, Nadine Stair, expressed this philosophy particularly well:

If I Had My Life to Live Over

I'd like to make more mistakes next time. I'd relax, I would limber up. I would be sillier than I have been this trip. I would take fewer things seriously. I would take more chances. I would climb more mountains and swim more rivers. I would eat more ice cream and less beans. I would perhaps have more actual troubles, but I'd have fewer imaginary ones.

You see, I'm one of those people who live sensibly and sanely hour after hour, day after day. Oh, I've had my moments, and if I had it to do over again, I'd have more of them. In fact, I'd try to have nothing else. Just moments, one after another, instead of living so many years ahead of each day. I've been one of those persons who never goes anywhere without a thermometer, a hot water bottle, a raincoat, and a parachute. If I had to do it again, I would travel lighter than I have.

If I had my life to live over, I would start barefoot earlier in the spring and stay that way later in the fall. I would go to more dances. I would ride more merry-go-rounds. I would pick more daisies.

Look, I really don't want to wax philosophic, but I will say that if you're alive, you got to flap your arms and legs, you got to jump around a lot, you got to make a lot of noise, because life is the very opposite of death. And therefore, as I see it, if you're quiet, you're not living. You've got to be noisy, or at least your thoughts should be noisy and colorful and lively.
—MEL BROOKS

MAKING THE MOST
OF THE TIME YOU HAVE LEFT

With a book title like *Living Positively* many people assume that this is a book about positive thinking. Well, it is and it isn't.

Certainly, as obvious as it sounds, the most important factor in being happy *is deciding to be happy*, regardless of what life challenges you may be faced with.

But it's not quite that simple. As we've said before, for those of us living with HIV/AIDS, everything is not necessarily wonderful all the time, and it can be very unhealthy to pretend that everything is fine when it's not. There is a fine line between "*focusing on the positive*," which is realistic and healthy, and the term "*positive thinking*," which to my mind can be a form of "denial" which is neither.

For example, if you were to cut yourself badly with a kitchen knife, the person who just *thinks positively* might think happy thoughts, pray or meditate, and affirm or visualize that all would be well. That person might also end up having bled to death on the kitchen floor. If you ignore something serious, it could get worse. Even symptoms can be good; they are the body's way of communicating with you.

The person who *focuses on the positive* might realistically see the situation as it is, and take some urgent action, getting bandages or going to the emergency room and getting proper medical attention. Now, in addition to this, they might focus on calm, healing thoughts, and on a positive outcome. They probably would feel better, might get more friendly and thorough service from the hospital staff, and maybe—just maybe—they might even heal faster.

Let's say you're lucky enough to go on a vacation in Hawaii. When you get back, all your friends want to hear every detail. You could tell them about how long the flight was, how you almost missed your connecting flight, how dirty the cab was from the airport, how crowded the first beach you went to was, etc., etc.

You could also tell them about how beautiful that first sunset was, how friendly the cab driver had been from the airport, how spectacular the beach had been on the second day, about all the truly friendly people you made friends with, etc., etc.

Both stories are equally true, but which would you rather hear? For some unknown reason, we all seem to fall into telling the "ain't it awful" story. Looking at the bright side does not mean that you pretend that everything is always perfect. Life doesn't work that way.

An optimist may see a light where there is none, but why must the pessimist always run to blow it out?

*MICHEL
DE SAINT-PIERRE*

I'm sure everyone has been asked "How are you today?" by someone who really wants to know. If you think about it long enough, each of us can find a long list of things that aren't so good today. The more we focus on this list of aches and pains, the worse we are going to feel. It's a rare day indeed where we can't find at least a few things that are pretty good today.

How are you today? Start out by searching for all things that are good, and make sure to include as many as you can think of. After you've finished that, you may include the things that perhaps aren't so wonderful, but don't dwell on them, or glorify telling the "ain't it awful" part of the story.

There's a story about another form of unhealthy "positive thinking" we might call "faith without action."

Once upon a time, there was this king who knew that God was with him. Before a great battle, a spy came to the king to sell battle secrets. Since the king knew that God was with him, he did not need to buy information, so he sent the spy away.

The next morning, the king was brought his mighty armor, but since the king knew that God was with him, he gave his armor away. In battle, although the king fought mightily, he was soon struck down and gravely wounded. A surgeon appeared, but again the king knew that God was with him, so he sent the doctor away.

The king died and went to heaven, where he asked God, "Why did you forsake me?" God replied "Forsake you? To stop the battle, first I sent you your enemy's secrets, then to protect you, I gave you mighty armor. Finally, to heal your wound, I sent a great surgeon. You turned down all my gifts, and here you are."

REINVENTING YOUR FUTURE

I think most of us, when we first start dealing with HIV/AIDS, greatly reduce our long-term plans for the future. Even if we don't think that we're going to get sick or die anytime soon, perhaps we spend a little more money enjoying today and put a little less away for our retirement.

This can be very bad indeed. Life is a lot like riding a bicycle: you tend to go in the direction that you're looking.

If we stop looking forward, then we have nothing to look forward to. If you spend too much time focusing on aches, pains, and all the other troubles, traumas, and tragedies in life, then you will almost certainly be able to find even more troubles, traumas, and tragedies.

A number of years ago, my mother was gravely ill: she spent over a hundred days in the hospital recovering from two heart attacks, two strokes, and having a good part of her heart replaced with plastic and metal. The doctors didn't give us much hope.

My mother had always loved to garden, so when she finally came back from the hospital, she wanted to plant for next season. Most people thought that this was pretty stupid. Certainly she would either be in a nursing home or dead before these flowers ever came up. But she insisted, and we humored her, and on her good days, we planted.

It was very important to her. She knew that the odds were stacked against her, but she needed to keep moving forward. That first winter, she was determined to see her flowers come up in the spring. She did. The next year, she gave up the burden of her old suburban house and moved into an easier to manage apartment in town. Of course, she immediately planted a new flower garden for her new home that is still the talk of the town.

He who has a why to live can bear almost any how.
—NIETZSCHE

That first Christmas, with all her problems and my HIV, we all knew that there was a very real possibility that one or both of us might not be around next Christmas. Since both of us were physically doing all right, we talked about it, and decided that we were going to make this the best Christmas ever.

I took time off from work to spend the day with her shopping and seeing the sights in New York City. Together we baked Christmas treats that she hadn't bothered with "since the children were small." We were determined to make some memories for her grandchildren (and my nieces and nephews).

Like most families, after my brother and sister got married and had families of their own, we had drifted apart. Well, this Christmas was going to fix all that. We were going to be a family again.

We made an old-fashioned Danish gingerbread house from scratch. We realized that to use all the ornaments that had accumulated we were going to need two trees, so naturally we bought even more ornaments and overstuffed an upstairs and a downstairs tree. A friend of mine said that my mother's house put the department stores to shame. And it did.

With all the love and effort that we both put in, sure enough it was the best Christmas ever. Oh, things weren't perfect: there were family rifts that took a few more years to heal, and none of us had the money that we used to, and the children behaved like children. But oh, what a Christmas that was!

The best part was that neither my mother nor I died the next year. At Christmas, we did it all again. I think objectively, it took us a couple of years to get it right again, but that first Christmas "back" will always stick in my mind.

It's important to keep dreaming of the future, keep planting our flower gardens for next year, and keep baking those cookies, and savoring the childlike wonder of each Christmas, regardless of how irrational this may seem to others.

Where do you see yourself next year? Five years from now? Twenty-five years from now? What about when you are one hundred years old? Be open to the wonderful possibilities.

It almost seems like a contradiction, but the more we live in the present and enjoy the moment, the farther our goals and dreams reach into the future. The more time we spend worrying about the future, the smaller our goals and dreams become.

Our society is big on delayed gratification. We're told that we should go to work every day even if we don't like our jobs, and we will be rewarded with two weeks off each year and once we reach a certain age we may "retire" and live off our lifelong savings.

Others spend so much time playing that they never have time to realize their dreams and they don't have any reserves to get them through the tough times.

It's like the fairy tale about the ant and the grasshopper. The grasshopper played all summer while the ant worked, and when the winter came, the grasshopper had no food or shelter. We need to make time to have fun in the moment while we balance out building the best future we can.

List at least a dozen activities that you enjoy doing, simply for the act of doing them. What do you find fun? What makes you laugh or smile? Schedule time to try these activities again.

Always leave enough time in your life to do something that makes you happy, satisfied, or even joyous. That has more of an effect on economic well-being than any other single factor.
—PAUL HAWKEN

YOU CAN DO WHAT YOU THINK YOU CAN DO

To illustrate how important one's attitude can be, let me give you an example. Let's say there are two identical groups of hikers on a difficult mountain trail. The previous season, the park rangers noticed that out of every ten hikers who started the trail, only two actually got all the way to the end. On average, eighty percent failed to finish the trail.

The first group's leader took each hiker aside, one by one, before they started. She told each one that she knew that they had what it takes, and were obviously one of the twenty percent that could master the trail. Although some of the group might not make it all the way, she asked that together they set a good pace and good example, and try to help the weaker hikers get as far as they can.

The second group's leader told all the hikers in his group that most of them wouldn't make it all the way, and when they did fall behind, they should turn back so as not to hold up the rest of the group.

Imagination is more important than knowledge.
—ALBERT EINSTEIN

Which of these two groups would you expect to have the higher percentage of success? The first, of course. These same ideas are true in living with HIV/ AIDS, or any other life-challenging condition.

HOW DO YOU KNOW WHAT'S GOOD NEWS?

There is a Taoist story about a poor man who lived alone with his son in an abandoned shack outside of a small village. Their only possession was a very old workhorse.

One day, the workhorse ran away. Hearing of

this, all the poor man's friends felt sorry for him: "That is so terrible for you," they said. The poor man simply answered, "How do you know?"

The next day the old workhorse returned, bringing with it a dozen young wild horses. Everyone in the town came by to see the poor man's miracle. "That is so wonderful for you," they all said. The poor man again answered, "How do you know?"

The day after that, the son tried to put one of these wild horses to work in the field. Being unused to wearing a harness, the horse kicked, and the son was badly injured. Again everyone said, "That is so terrible for you". Again the poor man simply answered, "How do you know?"

On the third day, a great army came through the village and forced all able-bodied young men to join them and fight in a great war from which few would ever return. The poor man's son was still too bruised to go.

By the next week, the son completely recovered, and, with a dozen young, strong workhorses, the man and his son became the richest family in town.

What makes something "terrible" or "wonderful"? Sometimes life's biggest heartbreaks crack open the shell we can build around our heart. After we go through all the pain—which isn't easy—we can be either more open, more loving, and more loved, or we can build up even more scar tissue and become more numb.

When one door of happiness closes another door opens; but often we look so long at the closed door that we do not see the one that has been opened for us.
—HELEN KELLER

Since we never know how things will turn out in the end until the end, we might as well act as if they are going to turn out best in the long run, even if we don't understand how or why. Then, if they do, we didn't waste any time or energy being unhappy about life's opportunities that are camouflaged as problems. If they don't, well at least we didn't make things that much worse by piling our worries and fears on top of an already bad situation.

It all boils down to how you choose to think about something. As strange as it may seem, there is really very little difference between the feeling of dread behind "Oh no, that's terrible!" and the feeling of excitement in "Oh boy, that's wonderful!"

YOU ARE NOT AVERAGE

Some people claim that, statistically speaking, people with AIDS will die within a few short years. But statistics can only show what happens to the mythical, mathematically "average" person. Luckily, you are not average, and in reality no one else is, either. I doubt if you are really average in any way at all. Chances are, you personally didn't earn exactly $19,841 in 1992, but this was the average income per adult in the United States according to the United States Department of Commerce.

The Department of Commerce says very little about what *your* income was; there are too many other factors involved. Some are obvious, such as whether you are employed, what your occupation is, what training and background you have, and where you live. For example, in some cities, the average income is almost four times that of many rural areas. Other factors can be even more important, but are less obvious. These include your ambitions, your attitude, your priorities, and your expectations. These all play a vital role in how well you do financially.

Let's take a look at averages and statistics. If we take a large enough group of people, say everyone who lives in the United States, we can pretty accurately predict how many of them will die each day. We could even figure out the average age that these people died. But all of these averages say nothing about when any one person is expected to die.

For example, let's say out of a large group of people with some hypothetical life-challenging disease, the mathematical averages indicate that 80% will die within ten years. Many "realistic" doctors will tell all 100% that they will probably be dead within ten years. Just like the example with average income, that doesn't say anything about you, and like the hiker example, many people who might have been able to make it, won't bother to try their hardest, since they believe that they will fail anyway.

Having faith that you just might be one of the twenty percent to beat this thing can make you push harder than you ever thought possible, and create remarkable results. It doesn't matter if the odds are one out of five or one out of a million, someone is going to be that one, and it might as well be you. As John-Roger and Peter McWilliams wrote in *You Can't Afford the Luxury of a Negative Thought*, "If anyone has ever beaten your disease before, so can you. If no one has, you can be the first."

YOU MAY BE THAT ONE-IN-A-MILLION

How much longer will you, or anyone, with HIV/AIDS live? Well, in the US "on average" about two years from being diagnosed with AIDS, but some people aren't diagnosed until they have almost died, and others might live a normal, healthy life for decades.

No one can ever predict how much longer anyone has on this planet. There is a very real possibility that TODAY could be the last day you are alive. The odds are, however, that you will live. TODAY just might be the very last day you have left. That's not very likely, but it could happen. You also might live until you are 120 (or older). Again, this isn't very likely, but it could happen. The odds are somewhere in between.

WE BELIEVE WHAT WE SAY AND HEAR

Words are very powerful things. What we say, and how we say it, has a profound impact on how we feel, and how we view ourselves.

Thoughts and emotions are very delicate things, and our subconscious tends to believe what we see, hear, and say. As children, didn't we all have nightmares from watching a scary movie? Our subconscious didn't understand that the monsters weren't real. The evening news can be even more terrifying for us today, because these monsters, to some degree, are real.

Louise Hay, the first megastar of the New Age movement, goes so far as to advise people never to watch TV news, read the paper, or anything else disturbing *in the evening,* because whatever you are thinking about just before bed you take into sleep with you. She suggests that you save these activities for the morning, when you can have the whole day to process them.

On some level, we really believe what we hear, particularly from ourselves. When we tell ourselves "I haven't gotten that symptom yet" we reinforce that we probably will someday. This is a very different message from "*I never* got that symptom."

Telling ourselves "I can't do such-and-such anymore," we close our mind to the possibility that we ever might again in the future, whereas saying "I haven't been able to do such-and-such so far" opens us to the challenge.

It may sound silly, but whenever I hear the shorthand "I am HIV," I shudder. We are so much more than just our bodies, and certainly not defined by some little virus that happens to be inside our body. HIV may be important, but certainly doesn't define who we are as a person.

The human spirit can't be diagrammed or dissected; it can't be seen by tomographic scanners and it can't be represented by numbers on a medical chart. Yet it is the single most identifiable feature of human uniqueness. Unless it is understood and respected, all other facts are secondary.
—NORMAN COUSINS

The words "I am . . ." are potent words; be careful what you hitch them to. The thing you're claiming has a way of reaching back and claiming you.
—A.L. KITSELMAN

THE "PROBLEM" WITH "SHOULD"

There are two words that, more than all the others, I wish were removed from the English language; they are "should" and "problem."

"Problems" are bad things, and as we've seen, one doesn't always know how things will turn out in the end. Often, the biggest difficulties are really the things we benefit from the most. Since we never know which is which, I like to label all of them "opportunities."

"Should" means that something is somehow required, or morally obligated. If you choose not to do it, then you are, to some degree, a bad person for not doing what you "should" have done. Perhaps it even makes you wrong or bad for not having done this thing already. "Should" is a word that is loaded with guilt and judgment, and limits your actions.

No matter how much you do, there is always something that you haven't done yet. Therefore, no matter how much you do, there is always something to feel guilty about.

Often, when we choose to do one thing we have labeled we "should" do, we can't do something else we have also labeled we "should" do. We end up feeling guilty for not doing the other one. It's like the joke about the mother who gives her son two neckties. He makes a big fuss and promptly puts one on. The mother looks rejected and says, "What, you didn't like the other one?"

Also, "should" is often used with "not." Not doing something is a lot of work. Those of us who have tried not drinking, not smoking, or not thinking about something know this. It's much easier to do something else than it is to not do something.

"Could," on the other hand, is a much more powerful, yet gentler word. It gives you choices, and doesn't make you wrong or bad if you choose to do something else.

When written in Chinese, the word "crisis" is composed of two characters. One represents danger and the other represents opportunity.

—JOHN F. KENNEDY

"Could" also opens the door to more than one alternative. If you "should" do something, then that is the only choice on the list. On the other hand, if you "could" do something, then the mind opens up a whole list of other things that you could also do. Now you have a choice; you have options.

Imagine that you say to yourself "I *should* do the laundry." Now, unless you spring to your feet, gather up the dirty towels, and rush to the nearest washing machine, there will probably be a little voice inside that says "Yes, but you're not doing it, are you? You lazy, good-for-nothing, always goofing off. No wonder your life is such a mess, you can't even get around to doing a simple thing like your laundry" and on and on.

Now let's replay that scene with you saying to yourself "I *could* do the laundry." Now you might say "Yes I could, but I also want to call some friends I haven't spoken to in a while, or I could catch up on my reading, or even my TV watching. Now let's see, what do I want to do most right now?"

Don't "should" on yourself or others. Each person who must cope in some way with HIV/AIDS will find their own way of doing so. What works for some people will not work for others. Sometimes this can be very frustrating when you see someone else who you think isn't coping with it in the "right way." Remember that there are no right or wrong ways, only options and alternatives.

Thinking is an experiment dealing with small quantities of energy, just as a general moves miniature figures over a map before setting his troops in action.
—SIGMUND FREUD

JUDGMENT WORDS

"Should" and "problem" are not the only words that carry with them some underlying judgments.

Although they are over a dozen years old, which is a very long time in the history of HIV/AIDS, "The Denver Principles," written by the People with AIDS Advisory Committee in June 1983, address some other labels particularly well:

We condemn attempts to label us as "victims," which implies defeat, and we are only occasionally "patients," which implies passivity, helplessness and dependence upon the care of others. We are "people with AIDS."

Really take a look at the words you use, and what they really are saying. For example, calling someone a "drug addict" labels that person as being bad, a "drug user" is nonjudgmental. "Innocent victim" suggests that someone else is guilty. The word "promiscuous" I like to define as meaning someone who has sex with one more partner than the person using the word. "Promiscuous" has a moralizing tone, when most of the time, people only mean sexually active.

Now that we've grounded ourselves in the present and gained momentum by enjoying the journey focusing on the positive, we're now ready to "take our show on the road" and reach out to others . . .

CHAPTER 5

HELPING OTHERS AND LETTING OTHERS HELP YOU

> 3   HIV/AIDS can be too tough and confusing to deal with alone. Luckily, you don't have to. You may be surprised how supportive friends, family, coworkers, and the rest of your community can be in helping you deal with all the everyday difficulties, errands, annoyances, contradictions, and fears.
>
> Regardless of how bad (or good) things might be for you, helping someone who's having a hard time—even if it's only reaching out to them with a phone call—will help you forget your own troubles and make you grateful for your good fortune. It also makes you both feel better. Remember how good it feels to help others, and give someone else that opportunity too, by sometimes letting others help you.

Independence and self-sufficiency is a myth. Everyone is dependent on everyone else. Who in the modern world actually grows their own food or builds their own shelter? And of those rare few who do, did they do so with the help of tools not of their own making or invention?

For some reason, as a society we believe in the myth of the lone, self-sufficient cowboy. We are told it is weak to ask for help. As children, many of us are taught that we should try to help others, but very few of us are taught how to ask for help for ourselves.

This is too bad, because that's just not the way

It is one of the most beautiful compensations of this life that no man can sincerely try to help another without also helping himself.
—*RALPH WALDO EMERSON*

it works. It takes a lot of courage to reach out, and groups such as Alcoholics Anonymous and cancer support groups have proven that "together we are able to do what none of us has been able to do individually."

One of the big changes brought on by living with HIV/AIDS is that people who have fostered the illusion of being strong and self-sufficient now must admit that they need help. They need other people in support groups, they need doctors, and sometimes they need help cleaning up their homes and doing laundry. Sometimes they need help financially.

Everybody wants to do something to help, but nobody wants to be first.
—PEARL BAILEY

Support groups are a wonderful place to get all this off your chest and get your emotional batteries charged. You can talk with others who have already gone through what you are going through, people who offer not only support but also practical advice on treatments and other programs.

They are also a great way to meet new friends and engage in social activities. Many people living with HIV/AIDS do not feel comfortable sharing all the details of their health status with members of their family, friends, and coworkers. Having a place to unwind and talk about these details can be very important.

Sometimes it's these well-meaning family members whom we need to get away from for a while. They "tidy up" our private things. Home health aides rearrange the bathroom so you can't find anything—it seems like the whole world knows your every move.

Sometimes, prejudice is like a hair across your cheek. You can't see it, you can't find it with your fingers, but you keep brushing at it because the feel of it is irritating.
—MARIAN ANDERSON

One of the reasons that HIV/AIDS groups work is that they offer a safe place to talk about these issues. Individual names and information that are offered at a meeting are not to be repeated outside that meeting. If you want to talk about what happened to someone who didn't attend that meeting, you can omit or invent names or other information that would indicate who was involved.

Meeting others and getting phone numbers is an important part of being a member of a support group. You have to live with HIV/AIDS one hundred and sixty-eight hours each week, and support groups generally last only one hour each week. That leaves one hundred and sixty-seven hours that can be pretty tough sometimes. Getting phone numbers *and calling* other people who are living with HIV/AIDS is an important part of reaching out.

 Make a list of at least twenty people (both men and women) who can be members of your support team. Go down the list and check in with at least two of them each day. That way, if you're ever having a hard time, you are in the habit of reaching out and talking with others.

One of the best things about support groups and AIDS service organizations is that beyond helping you, they offer you all sorts of opportunities for helping others.

Although this help makes the world a better place, it is also important for purely selfish reasons. A recovering alcoholic knows the best way to stay sober is to help other people get sober. The cure for helplessness and frustration is becoming part of the solution by helping others or through some form of political or social action. Too often we can focus on ourselves and our own very real problems. Reaching out to others lets us shift our focus and helps someone else in the process.

Having an upbeat attitude feels better than having a doom-and-gloom attitude. For a moment let's take a step back and instead of looking at what we can do to change things, let's look at what we can do to change the way we look at how things are.

Here are five good reasons to reach out and help others:

We live very close together. So, our prime purpose in this life is to help others. And if you can't help them, at least don't hurt them.
—THE DALAI LAMA

No man is an island, entire of itself; every man is a piece of the continent, a part of the main.
—JOHN DONNE

1. It offers a distraction from your own problems. On a purely escapist level, when you are focused on helping someone else, it doesn't give you much time to think about your own problems.

2. It's good for your self-esteem: it's easy to feel useless and helpless. Helping someone else proves that what you do really does make a difference.

3. If you help others when they need help, then others will be more likely to help you when you need help. It's like putting a little something away for a rainy day.

4. It can just plain feel good to watch someone else receive your help.

5. Most of the important stuff we learn in life is through trial and error, and those errors can be pretty painful. Helping others lets you learn about a whole slew of things before you have to.

The essence of our effort to see that every child has a chance must be to assure each an equal opportunity, not to become equal, but to become different—to realize whatever unique potential of body, mind, and spirit he or she possesses.

—JOHN FISCHER

There are all kinds of places to turn for help, including: local AIDS services organizations, programs at local health departments and colleges, employee assistance programs, HIV/AIDS support groups, twelve-step programs, support groups for cancer and other life-challenging conditions, gay and lesbian community centers (often with HIV/AIDS resources open to everyone, gay and straight), women's health centers, church and other organized religious programs, less traditional spiritual programs, healing centers of all kinds, and all sorts of extended families and friends who want to help.

Looking at "Appendix B: National and Regional Resources," you will find hundreds of organizations that are there to help. They are in every state and most major cities. Often, local doctors and organizations in nearby cities know about resources right in your neighborhood or town.

It's a pity we can't forget our troubles the same way that we forget our blessings.
—ALCOHOLICS ANONYMOUS

CHAPTER 6

DOING HEALTHY STUFF AND
AVOIDING UNHEALTHY STUFF

> 4 Do things that are healthy for your body, mind, and
> spirit, and avoid those that are not. Being healthy is about
> balance, variety, and moderation in all the aspects of your
> life. Learn to listen to your body; it may be trying to tell you
> something. Avoid focusing too much attention on any one
> small piece—you might be ignoring the larger whole.

CURING THE CAUSES,
NOT THE SYMPTOMS

In *The Power of Positive Thinking* Norman Vincent
Peale wrote that "Most people are as happy and
healthy as they choose to be." On some level, this is
certainly true.

I think most of us, in our hearts, already know
many of the things we need to do to be healthier. But
we all forget. Everyone knows *some actions* that are
healthy to do and other things that are not so healthy.

We know, for example, that eating proper
amounts of nutritious food, drinking plenty of fluids,
getting moderate exercise and rest is healthier than not
doing these things.

For those of us living with HIV/AIDS, we need all
the health that we can get. I'm sure that no one would
claim that being a coach potato, not getting enough
sleep, drinking too much alcohol, using too many "recreational" drugs, living on junk food, smoking too

*To keep the body in
good health is a
duty . . . otherwise
we shall not be able
to keep our mind
strong and clear.*
      —BUDDHA

56

many cigarettes, drinking too much caffeine, eating too much sugar, being under too much stress, or even being in unhealthy relationships is *healthier* for you than avoiding these things. Yet many of us, nevertheless, do not always choose the healthier options.

List ten activities that are currently part of your life that, if you were to reduce or quit, might help your body, mind, and spirit to be even healthier. Include those things that are so enjoyable that they are not worth letting go of at present.

List another ten activities that are not currently part of your regular program that you might consider adding to help your body, mind, and spirit to be even healthier.

Why don't we always choose the option that is healthiest for us in the long run? The reason is simple. For most people, most of the time, breaking "the rules" by choosing a less-healthy alternative has few consequences, at least for the short run. This is unfortunate, since the ill effects happen so long after the behavior that we forget. In the short run, most of us seem to be able to play without having to pay. In the long run, however, most of us not only have to pay, we pay with interest.

If, for example, you ate one strawberry, and as soon as it was in your mouth you became violently ill, you probably wouldn't eat many strawberries, no matter how much you loved the taste. Unfortunately, our bodies often don't give us such clear signs, and often the very things that destroy our bodies seem so enjoyable when we do them.

This mentality has not only caused us individual sickness, but created a sick society. So many of us want immediate, personal gratification, and don't seem to care about the long-term costs. We avoid asking "What does this really cost us in the long run?"

We all have a lot to learn from the Native Amer-

There is little sense in attempting to change external conditions, you must first change inner beliefs, then outer conditions will change accordingly.
—BRIAN ADAMS
How to Succeed

icans, who traditionally considered the effects their actions would have on their great-great-great-great-grandchildren. Imagine what our society would be like if we focused on what is best for our joint future rather than our personal profits this quarter. What would happen to our national debt, the global environment, the inner cities, and leveraged buyouts?

For those of us living with HIV/AIDS, it is particularly important to listen to our bodies and to try to heal *the cause* of our problems. Many of us spend more time, energy, and money taking care of replaceable things, such as our cars, homes, or even our clothes, than we do our bodies.

Frequently, the little effort we spend on our bodies is focused on looking good rather than being truly healthy. Being healthy means more than just being symptom-free. In our society, we view symptoms as being somehow unrelated to their causes.

Whenever we experience a problem—anything from indigestion to a heart attack—too many of us simply run to our local drugstore or doctor to get a quick fix. We ask for something that removes the symptoms without requiring too much effort on our part, even if this "fix" doesn't address what may have caused the problems in the first place. This is a pity, because symptoms are good: they are the body's way of telling us that something is out of balance.

Those indigestion relief commercials on TV are a perfect example. The ads tell us that if we are in pain from eating unhealthy food, too much stress, or other bad habits, we should buy some pills, and—plop, plop, fizz, fizz—we will feel fine. Through the wonders of modern technology we can keep damaging our body for a while longer. This is like disconnecting the warning light in your car rather than adding oil.

How many people would prefer their doctor to tell them that they might just be experiencing the re-

We grew up founding our dreams on the infinite promise of American advertising. I still believe that one can learn to play the piano by mail and that mud will give you a perfect complexion.

—ZELDA FITZGERALD Save Me the Waltz

sults of a poor diet, lack of proper exercise, and that if they would change their life-style, they might be healthier? Although it's easier to take some new pill, often the best answers are within ourselves.

YOU ARE WHAT YOU PUT INTO YOUR BODY

The single largest factor in your health is what you put into your body—food, drugs, and other chemicals.

The body is a living machine. It needs energy to operate, and that energy comes from burning (really oxidizing or metabolizing) the fuel content of food or the energy reserves that our body has stored away for a rainy day, which we call body fat. The amount of energy stored in food—or anything else for that matter—is measured in calories.

We get this energy from three types of foods:

1. *Carbohydrates*, such as sugars and starches that are produced by plants. These have 4 calories of energy per gram, or about 1,800 calories per pound. Most of our energy comes from carbohydrates.
2. *Proteins* come from meat, fish, dairy, and some plants when eaten in the proper combinations. They also have 4 calories of energy per gram.
3. *Fats* such as oil, butter, and animal fats contain about twice as much energy, just over 9 calories per gram, or about 4,000 calories per pound.

In addition to our energy needs, the body must repair itself. Fortunately, the body is able to manufacture most of the chemicals and cells that it needs, but it does need some basic raw materials to be able to do this. These raw materials are as follows:

To laugh often and much; to win the respect of intelligent people and the affection of children; to earn the appreciation of honest critics and endure the betrayal of false friends; to appreciate beauty; to find the best in others; to leave the world a bit better, whether by a healthy child, a garden patch, or a redeemed social condition; to know even one life had breathed easier because you have lived. This is to have succeeded.
—RALPH WALDO EMERSON

- *Proteins* are both an energy source and one of the raw materials needed to build and rebuild the body.

- *Vitamins* are organic, meaning that they are obtained from plants and animals.

- *Minerals*, such as calcium, iron, potassium, sodium, or zinc, are inorganic, meaning that they were originally obtained from rocks.

In addition to these nutrients, scientists have identified more than 40 other nutrients that are required for good health. Since no single food, or even type of food, can supply all these—plus the dozens more that probably are needed that we don't yet know about—it's important to eat a wide variety of foods.

PLENTY OF WATER AND FIBER

A wise man should consider that health is the greatest of human blessings, and learn how by his own thought to derive benefit from his illness.

—HIPPOCRATES

Lastly, the human body is over 80% water, and all of the reactions necessary for life use water. The body needs to get rid of toxins and the waste after the energy and raw materials have been removed from the food. For this, we need *plenty of water* to flush out all the toxins from the internal organs and *enough fiber or bulk* to keep the digestive system moving.

For people living with HIV/AIDS, dehydration can easily result from difficulty swallowing, lack of thirst, diarrhea, fatigue, excessive perspiration, or many other factors.

There is also increased need for more water because of the increased levels of toxic substances generated during the immune response itself as well as toxic by-products from medications and supplements that need to be flushed from the body.

Although each person's needs are different, a good rule of thumb is that every day, each person should drink at least sixty-four ounces of water, which is the same as about eight large glasses, or about two liter or quart bottles.

THE ANTI-AIDS DIET MIRACLE

There have been more best-selling books about what and how to eat than on any other subject. Everything from cookbooks to the latest fad diets line the shelves of every bookstore. Unfortunately, no two seem to agree on exactly what the "right" things are.

The more books you read, the more seminars you attend, and the more "experts" you consult with, the more confusing and elusive the answers seem to be. To make things even worse, few of these books and studies were done with the needs of someone living with HIV/AIDS in mind. Please see in "Appendix A: Suggested Reading" the section on *Holistic Treatment and Nutritional Therapy* for some of the very best resources in this area.

Although there is a great deal of sound advice out there, the world is filled with nutritional quacks who will try to sell you their latest diet, supplement, or "health food." Some of these people are outright con artists, others well-meaning but underinformed people.

Just because a person is a "board-certified doctor," doesn't mean that he or she knows what's best for you. Be particularly careful of anyone who is trying to sell you anything—even in doctor's offices or health food shops. These "salespeople" are often only given information that sells whatever they have to sell. Avoid all-in-one miracles where a single food or supplement is the magic cure-all, and you can continue to eat whatever you want. Healthy nutrition—like life—is about balance, variety, and moderation.

BODY FAT

Most Americans weigh more than is healthy for them, and everyone seems to be obsessed with losing weight.

No permanent healing is possible if a person continues to make the same mistake and thus invites the return of the disease.
—PARAMAHANSA YOGANANDA

Because of this, everything from TV talk shows to fast-food restaurants feature "good nutrition," "eating right," and "healthy foods," when they really mean "low in calories" or "to promote weight loss."

Our image of what is "healthy" is colored by this obsession. Most of us think we "should" look like the men and women in the underwear ads. This may be what is fashionable, but it is not necessarily what is most healthy for people living with HIV/AIDS.

From time to time, almost everyone, regardless of HIV/AIDS, gets sick and is laid up in bed for a number of days. If you are unable to eat enough, your body starts to draw on its reserves—your fat layer—at just over 9 calories per gram, or about 4,000 calories per pound.

If you have one of those bodies without an ounce of fat (which is really about 6% body fat), then your body has to metabolize lean body mass, meaning muscle. This is far more difficult for your body to do, and it generates far more toxins in the process. The result is that the body has even more that it must recover from.

Although it might not be the most fashionable option, it's probably far healthier to be 10 to 15 pounds over your ideal weight, or something like 12% body fat. Weighing much more than this is not healthy either, since that taxes your body even more, and can lead to heart disease and other conditions that are significantly complicated by HIV/AIDS.

EATING RIGHT

Most of what you—and well-meaning family and friends—may have learned in the past about what and how to eat was probably about limiting calories and reducing cholesterol. If you are HIV-positive, these are probably not your main goals right now. You are probably much more concerned with improving general health, boosting the immune function, and extending longevity than you are with losing weight.

In addition to these goals, HIV/AIDS can add all sorts of specialized complications which, combined with side effects from various treatments, cause loss of appetite, difficulty swallowing, difficulty in the body absorbing and processing the food that has been eaten, and a number of digestive problems, including nausea, diarrhea, indigestion, and gas.

Your number one goal is to do whatever you have to do to avoid malnutrition or dehydration and maintain lean body mass and 12% body fat, even if you have to work on this every five minutes all day long.

A STRICT MACROBIOTIC, VEGETARIAN DIET

One persistent myth is that a strict macrobiotic, vegetarian diet is the best choice for living with HIV/AIDS. Unfortunately, this is not true. Certainly the typical American diet is far from the healthiest choice. Although macrobiotics are much healthier *in some respects for some people* than the typical American diet, it is certainly not a cure-all. If it were, by now we'd see whole groups of long-term survivors swear by it. This isn't the case.

A strict macrobiotic, vegetarian diet includes many foods and ingredients that are unfamiliar to many people, and can be too restrictive for some of the special needs of people with HIV/AIDS. Certainly no way of eating can work for anyone who doesn't like the food or who does not follow the plan.

What many people call "macrobiotic" is really just natural: whole grains, fresh vegetables and fruits and other organic foods that together constitute a high-protein, low-fat diet. I think most people—even the USDA—would agree this is generally healthier for most everyone.

Probably the most significant area of disagree-

If I can't dance, I don't want to be part of your revolution.

—EMMA GOLDMAN

ment is the role of animal protein, such as meats, poultry, or fish.

One school of thought is that since people with HIV/AIDS have difficulty absorbing protein from what they have eaten, vegetable proteins are too difficult to absorb, so they need to eat about 1 gram of animal protein per pound of body weight per day. That's about two large 6-oz cans of tuna fish each day for a 170-pound person.

The other school of thought is that this is so much more animal protein than is needed that it greatly taxes the body to process it. This second viewpoint is that complex vegetable proteins are *far more easily* absorbed than their animal alternatives.

The end result is something of a moving target. Foods and even whole methods of preparing foods may work effectively for quite some time, and then no longer work for you. The important thing is aggressively to seek out what works for you at present.

Do or do not. There is no "try."
—YODA

THE USDA "FOOD GUIDE PYRAMID"

The United States Department of Agriculture (USDA) has worked hard at establishing a good general purpose nutrition plan for the average American. This was certainly not designed for people with HIV/AIDS, but it does give a good mainstream starting point for finding what may be right for you.

To get your own copy of this guide, please see in "Appendix A: Suggested Reading" the section on *Holistic Treatment and Nutritional Therapy.*

The USDA's seven general dietary goals are:

1. Eat a variety of foods.
2. Maintain healthy weight.
3. Choose a diet that is low in fat, saturated fat, and cholesterol.
4. Choose a diet with plenty of vegetables, fruits, and grain products.

5. Use sugars only in moderation.
6. Use salt and sodium only in moderation.
7. If you drink alcoholic beverages, do so in moderation.

The term "pyramid" comes from their graphic representation of what foods to eat.

- At the point are fats, oils, and sweets, meaning that they should only be used sparingly.
- The next layer down includes milk, yogurt, and cheese (2–3 servings daily) and meat, poultry, fresh, dry beans, eggs, and nuts (2–3 servings).
- The middle layer is vegetables (3–5 servings) and fruit (2–4 servings).
- On the base is bread, cereals, rice, and pasta (6–11 servings)

One target for a well-balanced diet might be:

- 50 to 55% of calories from carbohydrates (mainly complex carbohydrates).
- 15 to 20% of calories from protein.
- 30% or less of calories from fat.

For example, a 2,800 calorie diet might include:

- 1,450 calories (365 grams) of carbohydrates (52%).
- 560 calories (140 grams) of protein (20%).
- 800 calories (89 grams) of fat (28%).

Begin with the possible; begin with one step. There is always a limit; you cannot do more than you can. If you try to do too much, you will do nothing.
—P.D. OUSPENSKY AND G.I. GURDJIEFF

YOUR PERSONAL FOOD PLAN

With all this contradictory information, it's easy to get confused into inaction. Unless you have a clear idea of what your "Food Plan" is, it's not likely that you will be able to follow it.

Write down your own personal "Food Plan." How much of what do you plan to eat each day? What foods do you want to avoid or limit? How will you keep track? How will you know if this is working for you?

FOOD SAFETY

Although HIV cannot be transmitted through food, people with HIV/AIDS (like older people, people with cancer, or others with lower immune functions) are in some cases 300 times more susceptible to some forms of "food poisoning" than the general population.

Not only are people with HIV/AIDS more likely to get food poisoning, the diseases that these infections cause can be far more serious for someone living with HIV/AIDS than they would be otherwise. They may even be fatal.

Food poisoning is caused by food-borne microorganisms, and almost all food poisoning comes from improperly prepared animal products, and can be prevented by following a few guidelines. Since it is almost impossible to tell what animal products are actually infected with disease-causing microorganisms, *all animal products must be treated as if they were infected.*

The two most important steps to avoid food poisoning are to *fully cook all animal products* and to be *very careful about personal and kitchen hygiene* by washing everything before, during, and after preparing food.

Remember that when anything comes in contact with any raw or undercooked animal products it *may become infected* and can transmit that infection. For example, if you handle fish with your hands or cut chicken on a cutting board and do not scrub these carefully afterward, the disease-causing microorganisms may be transferred to, say, vegetables that you might not be cooking enough to kill off these microorganisms.

Some particular things to be careful of are:

Remember, Ginger Rogers did everything Fred Astaire did, but she did it backwards and in high heels.
—FAITH WHITTLESEY

- Never eat any raw or undercooked meat, poultry, fish, or eggs. Cooking thoroughly kills off any infections.

- Never drink raw or unpasteurized milk, or eat milk products such as cheese made from raw or unpasteurized milk.

- When buying raw meat, poultry, or fish in the market, be very careful about any handling and storage. Even in the market, double-wrap packages in plastic bags so any drippings don't get on your fresh vegetables or other food in your cart or refrigerator.

- Wash and refrigerate all vegetables.

- Never leave meat, poultry, or fish (either cooked or uncooked) unrefrigerated.

- Check "sell by" dates to make sure everything is at its freshest.

- Check store displays and general cleanliness of stores and restaurants. When in doubt, walk out.

- When shopping, buy your nonperishable goods first, and go straight home after buying your raw meat, poultry, or fish, so they will spend the shortest possible time without refrigeration.

- Avoid eating animal products from street vendors, or other places where food might not have been kept either hot enough or cold enough.

- Be extremely careful in foreign countries where health codes are not as strict as they are in the US.

"RECREATIONAL" DRUGS

On a low level, the body has its own intelligence and knows how to stay in balance and to heal itself. Unfortunately, we humans like to impose our own ideas of how we want the body to behave by taking drugs of all kinds.

Perhaps when you think of "drugs" you think of crack cocaine in some burned-out building in the ghetto, some junkie shooting up heroin, or smoking marijuana at a rock concert.

Many readers will be surprised to learn how very general and nonspecific the word "drugs" is, depending on which legal definition you choose. In general, a drug is any nonnutritional substance that affects the body or central nervous system and causes some change in behavior.

By this definition, alcohol, nicotine (cigarettes), and caffeine (coffee, tea, and soda) can all be defined as being *drugs* and since they do not serve any therapeutic purpose, they are *"recreational"* drugs.

As anyone who has ever tried to quit smoking cigarettes, longed for that morning cup of coffee, or attended an AA meeting knows, all of these can also be *highly addictive* recreational drugs.

I know many readers will comment "surely this guy isn't suggesting that sipping a cup of *cappuccino* is just as bad as smoking a crack pipe?"

Of course I'm not. But "bad" is a moral judgment, and it's not my job to counsel anyone on morality. Like HIV/AIDS, drug use is not a moral question; it is a health issue. Probably moderate use of most drugs, for most people, is not too unhealthy, although total abstinence is unquestionably more healthy. The problem is when drug use crosses the line into being a bad habit or addiction.

The rule of thumb I use is, if the total cost in the long run—including financial and health effects—is smaller than the enjoyment, then you're fine. Have fun. If when you look back, it wasn't worth the long-term cost, then stop doing it. If you have trouble stopping, then it has become a bad habit or addiction, and is something you might want to look at seriously, or even get professional help with, or attend a twelve-step support group for.

Habit is habit, and not to be flung out of the window, but coaxed downstairs a step at a time.
—MARK TWAIN

Remember, the health effects and relative costs are different for people living with HIV/AIDS. Although 25% of the adult population smokes regularly, cigarettes are particularly dangerous for people with HIV/AIDS because respiratory complications are the number one cause of death for people with HIV/AIDS, and *smoking cigarettes halves the statistical life expectancy for people with HIV/AIDS.* That's a very high cost for not a lot of benefit. As important as quitting cigarettes can be, it is extremely difficult, since cigarettes can be even more addictive than cocaine or heroin.

One is too many, because one thousand isn't enough.
—ALCOHOLICS ANONYMOUS

 What recreational drugs do you use? Which ones are still worth all their costs, and which ones are just bad habits or addictions?

EXERCISE AND REST
Our bodies need exercise and rest every day. When most people think about exercise, they think about going to the gym so they can look a certain way. It's far more important how healthy *you are*, not how healthy *you look*.

The specifics naturally depend on the abilities of the individual person. The physical capabilities of people with HIV/AIDS range from world-class athletes to those unable to sit up in bed. Regardless of your current level of health, it's important to have an appropriate level of physical exercise to build your aerobic stamina, increase your energy level, build moderate muscle tone, reduce physical tension, and gain flexibility.

Resting in bed causes muscles to atrophy. Use it or lose it. If at all possible, get out of bed and sit in a chair. If you can do that, try walking with help. After that, perhaps build up to walking laps around the hospital floor. It might not be very interesting, but it will sure make you a lot healthier when you get out.

A general rule of thumb is that the "average healthy person" should get 30 minutes of aerobic activity three times a week. Aerobic exercise is any activity that increases the heart rate (and therefore the breathing rate) to a certain recommended level, and keeps it at this level for an extended period, usually at least 15 minutes. Many people may need to build up slowly to this prescribed 15 minutes. Personally, I strive for 45 minutes of aerobic activity five times a week.

Rest is a little more tricky. If you ever look at babies, they sleep all the time. That's because they need to. Their bodies have a lot of work to do. Sometimes, so do ours. On the other hand, sometimes we sleep because we want to hide from life. Only you can know which is which.

For fast-acting relief, try slowing down.
—LILY TOMLIN

Some healthy people need eight or nine hours every night, some can make do with only six or less. The important thing is to make sure you get what you need. The last thing you need is needlessly to run down your body just because you didn't give it the sleep it needed.

Sometimes, even when you've gotten a full night's sleep, you may feel tired. If so, rest some more. Your body usually knows what it's doing. Rather than pushing along at half speed for the rest of the day, a one-hour nap can be invigorating.

If you lose your possessions, you've lost a lot. If you lose your health, you've lost a great deal. But if you lose your peace of mind, you've lost everything.
—ANONYMOUS

CHAPTER 7

BECOMING YOUR OWN MEDICAL EXPERT

5 "Knowledge is Power." In an ideal world, your doctor and the rest of your health-care team would devote all their skills and energy to you. But try as they might, they have hundreds (or even thousands) of other patients and other conditions to keep up with. You have a much smaller case-load, and you can—if you really do your homework—know more about your personal condition than any doctor or other expert could.

Healing is a basic human function; not a medical touch or supernatural power.
—ANONYMOUS

To be able to make your own informed choices re-garding your health care, you don't need to know more than the doctors do, you just need to know enough to be able to carry on an intelligent conver-sation, and be able to ask the right questions. In the next chapter we will discuss some techniques for doing this.

In this chapter, we will look at some of the ter-minology, background information, medical facts, and theories one needs to understand when treating HIV/ AIDS. We'll look at how our bodies usually heal them-selves so you can get an idea how the pieces fit to-gether. You will also need to be able to understand the specialized medical language—or at least not be too confused or embarrassed when you don't.

EARLY HISTORY OF HIV/AIDS

Scientists can prove that HIV/AIDS has existed in humans for at least thirty-five years, and the evidence suggests that it probably has been around for over one hundred years, although it was not until 1981 that it became so widespread as to be studied.

Back in 1959, an otherwise healthy British sailor died from Pneumocystis carinii pneumonia (PCP) and other secondary or opportunistic infections (OIs) that are normally curable and only occur as symptoms of some other more serious, primary illness. However, in this sailor's case, there was no identifiable condition that might have caused these infections. Because of the mystery surrounding this death, Sir Robert Platt, the president of the Royal College of Physicians in England, personally supervised the autopsy and preserved samples from the sailor's body for later study. Sir Robert wrote in the medical record that he feared that "this might be the arrival of a new type of viral threat to the human species." How right he was!

Faced with the choice between changing one's mind and proving there is no need to do so, almost everyone gets busy on the proof.
—JOHN KENNETH GALBRAITH

In 1968, a fifteen-year-old boy from St. Louis, Missouri, was admitted to a hospital with unexplainable opportunistic infections including the rare skin cancer, Kaposi's sarcoma, but no identifiable primary disease. The boy died shortly thereafter, and again, because of the mystery of this case, tissue and fluid samples were frozen for later study.

In 1990, researchers reexamined many old medical records looking for early AIDS-like cases, and were able to detect the HIV virus in these early samples. Almost certainly, both the sailor and the boy had been infected for a number of years before their deaths. In an unrelated, but similar case also from 1959, another sample of blood from Zaire, Africa, tested HIV-positive.

Of course, no one can say how many other unexplained or misdiagnosed cases might have been HIV/

AIDS, particularly in less-developed countries where medical records were not so complete. Researchers have found published reports of AIDS-like outbreaks from 1902 to 1911, when a cluster of seven Italian men died from unexplained opportunistic infections. Between 1912 and 1966, there were another twenty-two cases throughout Europe and the Americas. In the sixties and seventies, outbreaks were even more numerous, beginning in equatorial Africa and reaching into central Africa, and eventually North America and Europe.

He who wonders discovers that this is in itself a wonder.
—M.C. ESCHER

The question one must ask is: "If HIV/AIDS has been around for so long, why hasn't it been a significant problem before, and why has it only recently become an epidemic?"

As we will discuss later in this chapter, unlike previous epidemics, HIV/AIDS is, luckily, very difficult to transmit: it requires direct, internal exposure to infected blood, semen, or vaginal lubrication. Only in the last few decades have we had just the right combination of factors that would allow this to happen: widespread use of blood transfusions and hypodermic needles, global air travel, sexual freedom, and the eradication of other "competing" diseases.

In order to protect the public health, the federal Centers for Disease Control (CDC) keeps track of outbreaks of illness from various health hazards. These range from the known diseases such as measles, tuberculosis, gonorrhea, syphilis, and even food poisoning, to relatively new threats such as Legionnaire's disease, toxic shock syndrome, and AIDS. The CDC uses specialized doctors, called epidemiologists, who act like medical detectives to try to find out what contributed to each outbreak and what might be done to prevent its spread or return in the future.

AIDS: ACQUIRED IMMUNE
DEFICIENCY SYNDROME

Beginning in the late seventies in New York, San Francisco, and Los Angeles, a number of people started being diagnosed with unusual, repeated infections and rare forms of cancer. Frequently these people died as a result of these usually minor conditions that the body generally could have healed by itself. Most of these first documented US cases (but not all) happened to be sexually active gay and bisexual men.

By June 1981, the United States Centers for Disease Control (CDC) formally described this syndrome, or collection of related diseases. A few weeks later, the *New York Times* published the now famous headline "Rare Cancer Seen In 41 Homosexuals." Even at this early date, doctors were guessing that this unnamed and unexplained condition was probably caused by some unknown virus that was sexually transmitted like the disease hepatitis B, which had been widely studied in the American gay community. By the end of 1981 there had already been 379 cases.

As we will discuss later in this chapter, whatever causes AIDS can be transmitted through sexual activity (homosexual or heterosexual), exposure to infected blood, and can be transmitted from mother to baby. Luckily, it cannot be transmitted through any casual or indirect means. Unfortunately, since the process may take many years or longer before any symptoms occur, a person could unknowingly infect many other potentially untraceable people before he or she becomes aware of his or her situation. This poses a unique public health problem.

At first the press called this "gay cancer" or "GRID" for Gay-Related Immune Deficiency. In Washington, Ronald Reagan had just come to power, and the newly elected conservative Republican administration was reluctant to focus on anything gay-

Two dejected assistants of Thomas Edison said:

"We've just completed our seven hundredth experiment and we still don't have the answer. We have failed."

"No, my friends, you haven't failed" replied Mr. Edison. "It's just that we know more about this subject than anyone else alive. And we're closer to finding the answer, because now we know seven hundred things not to do. Don't call it a mistake. Call it an education."

—SUSAN HAYWARD

related. This unfortunate consequence has had a far-reaching impact on the history of HIV/AIDS.

Increasingly, AIDS was discovered in hemophiliacs and transfusion recipients who received infected medical products made from blood. By June 1982, the more neutral name "AIDS" for Acquired Immune Deficiency Syndrome was uniformly adopted.

HIV: HUMAN IMMUNODEFICIENCY VIRUS

It took two years of research, but by 1983 Doctor Luc Montagnier's team from the Pasteur Institute in France first isolated the virus that most experts now consider to be primarily responsible for AIDS. In the United States, however, Robert Gallo from National Institutes of Health (NIH) also announced the same discovery. Although some scientists have questioned Gallo's procedures, Montagnier and Gallo officially now share the credit, and the neutral name Human Immunodeficiency Virus or HIV was chosen. Today, there is still a great deal of research as to the exact role HIV plays in the progression of AIDS, as we will discuss later in this chapter.

By March 1985, there had been such an outcry from those at risk of being infected by blood products that new laws were passed in the United States requiring that all blood products be tested for HIV antibodies. This, in addition to very strict medical sterilization procedures, has meant very few cases since then of people being infected through medical procedures such as blood transfusions, transplants, and other operations.

To avoid criticism, do nothing, say nothing, be nothing.
—ELBERT HUBBARD

In the United States, the risk of getting a unit of HIV-infected blood is now less than 1 in 300,000. Unfortunately, this is not also true in less-developed countries, where lack of financial resources limits the quality of medical resources, care, and testing.

WHO IS AFFECTED BY HIV/AIDS?

Unfortunately, in today's world everyone is affected in some way by HIV/AIDS. HIV affects men and women, gays and straights, the young and the old, the rich and the poor, addict and nonaddict, from practically every race, religion, ethnic origin, and life-style. It is spreading to every country and community on this planet, from the biggest, most metropolitan cities to the smallest rural villages.

In the early years of the AIDS epidemic, most of the people who were diagnosed with AIDS were gay men, injection drug users, prostitutes, and people from developing nations such as Haiti. Why HIV/AIDS hit these pockets of the population was merely an accident of history.

Unfortunately, this gave many people the mistaken impression that if they weren't part of one of these "high-risk groups," and didn't have sex with someone who was, they were pretty safe.

There is no such thing as a "high-risk group" for getting infected with HIV, there are only high-risk behaviors. Studies have been unable to show any one ethnic or social group that is more or less susceptible to HIV infection or progressing to AIDS than any other.

Because AIDS first emerged in the United States in the gay community, there has been a great deal of shame, secrecy, and gossip. In other parts of the world, however, the virus has been spread primarily through heterosexual contact. According to an estimate from the World Health Organization (WHO) in 1991, 3 out of 4 adults with HIV/AIDS worldwide were infected through heterosexual sex. This compares with only about 1 out of 16 adults in the United States with HIV/AIDS who were infected through heterosexual sex during the same time period.

For a number of reasons, it is difficult to know exact numbers. According to the Global AIDS Policy

Who Gets HIV?

What does the H in HIV stand for? Not homosexual Nor hemophiliac, Not Haitian, Nor heroin, Nor hypodermic needle. It stands for "Human." There are no high-risk groups, only high-risk behaviors.
—ALAN BARNETT

Coalition, about 19.5 million people worldwide were infected by the end of 1992. The International AIDS Center at Harvard estimated that of those, 7 million are in sub-Saharan Africa. Uganda, Africa, has been one of the hardest hit areas, with more than 1 out of every 10 people in the general population—and more than 1 out of every 3 women of childbearing age—being infected with HIV.

The most responsible estimates from the Eighth International AIDS Conference are that 40 million to more than 110 million people will have been infected with HIV by the year 2000. The number could be as high as about 1 out of every 50 people worldwide. Another person is infected with HIV every 15 seconds. Women now account for 40% of AIDS cases; 10% are children born to infected mothers.

In the United States estimates are that perhaps 2 million people have been infected with HIV. That's 1 out of every 125 men, women, and children in this country. To put this in perspective, there are more people living with HIV right now than there are police officers and security guards in this country.

According to the Centers for Disease Control (CDC) another American is diagnosed with AIDS every 6 minutes. There have been over 500,000 Americans diagnosed with AIDS, and almost 300,000 are already dead. Some say the actual numbers are much greater. Even so, this is many more Americans than were killed in battle during the Revolutionary, 1812, Mexican, Civil, Spanish-American, World War I, Korean, Vietnam, and Gulf wars combined.

In the cities, the problem is even worse. More than 1 out of 5 cases of AIDS in the US have been in the New York City area where AIDS is the leading cause of death for women of childbearing age. In Chelsea, one of Manhattan's hardest hit neighborhoods so far, about 3½%, or 1 out of every 30 adults, has been

Though people with disabilities have become more vocal in recent years, we still constitute a very small minority, yet the Beautiful People—the slender, fair, and perfect ones—form a minority that may be even smaller.

—DEBRA KENT

diagnosed with AIDS. It's staggering to think how many more must be HIV-positive.

In this country, 20% of all those diagnosed with AIDS were probably infected during their adolescence, and AIDS is now the sixth leading cause of death for all people 15 to 24 years old. According to the Urban Institute of Washington, DC, the majority of all adolescents in this country have had sex by the time they are seventeen, and most of those did so without using condoms regularly.

HIV IS THE VIRUS
THAT "CAN LEAD TO" AIDS

Why do some people with HIV get very sick and die so quickly, despite the best care, while others stay healthy for many, many years even though they might not take care of themselves at all? Why do some people become HIV-positive after only being exposed one time, and others can be exposed many times each day for many years and remain HIV-negative?

Some people have been frequently exposed to HIV for a long period of time—for example the wife or lover of someone who doesn't know that he or she is HIV-positive—and they remain HIV-negative. Others are exposed to only a tiny amount of virus only one time, and become infected. There are those who are HIV-positive that rapidly develop AIDS and die, and there are others who remain symptom-free for years, and might remain that way for the rest of their lives.

Lots of times you have to pretend to join a parade in which you're not really interested in order to get where you're going.
—GEORGE MORLEY

Today, there is still controversy over HIV. The question is really, "Does HIV cause AIDS?" Or to put it another way, "Is the HIV virus the single cause of AIDS?"

Well, the answer is either "probably yes" or "definitely not" depending on exactly what you mean by the question. Although the prevailing medical opinion is that the HIV "causes" AIDS, there is a vocal minority—who may be right—who believe that a great deal more research needs to be done. This may surprise some readers who have listened for years to the media describe HIV as "the AIDS virus."

Although we still don't have a complete picture of exactly how the HIV virus works and all the factors that are involved with AIDS, we do know that everyone who has AIDS also has been infected with HIV. The HIV virus—and perhaps some other mystery factors—can be transmitted through sexual contact or direct, internal exposure to infected blood, semen, vaginal fluid, spinal fluid, breast milk, or transplanted organs. HIV cannot be transmitted—although these other factors sometimes can be—through casual or less-direct contact, as we will discuss later in this chapter in the section on transmission.

The physician should know the invisible as well as the visible man. There is a great difference between the power which removes the invisible cause of disease and that which merely causes external effects to disappear.

—PARACELSUS

The problem is that the word "causes" means something very specific that is different from "is related to" or "may lead to." Saying "HIV causes AIDS" means that if people are not infected with HIV, they cannot get AIDS (true), and that if they are infected, they will always get AIDS (almost certainly not true).

To prove this in the laboratory, one would need to test everyone with AIDS and look for the HIV virus (this is easy, and has largely been done) and one would have to take a large number of healthy people that represented a cross section of the population, and infect half of them with HIV and the other half with some other virus, and wait until all of those infected with HIV got AIDS and see that none of those who were not infected with HIV ever got AIDS. Of course, you wouldn't be able to let them out of the laboratory for the rest of their lives, because that might introduce other factors. . . . Needless to say, since this analysis cannot be done, doctors look at a large enough group of people who are HIV-positive and see that a large percentage do eventually get AIDS (although many have not yet) and decide that the rest eventually will as well.

The other reason that it is difficult to say that HIV is the sole cause is that some of the diseases associated with AIDS, CMV and toxoplasmosis for example, are caused by other viruses. Many people in the general population have been infected with these viruses, but because they have strong immune systems which are able to fight off these diseases, they can live carrying these other viruses and never notice it. But those whose immune systems have been badly damaged by HIV cannot fight off these diseases. The important part is, if someone was never exposed to this other virus in the first place, it would not be possible to ever get that particular opportunistic infection.

Aside from these "cofactors," there are basic differences both in people and in the viruses that they are exposed to. Each person, animal, or microorganism inherits various strengths and weaknesses in the genetic code from its "parents."

In people we call this "genetic predisposition." Some people are able to become star football players or concert pianists, and others just aren't, no matter how much wonderful training they get, or how early you start training them. Some people are not allergic to poison ivy, and others can die from a bee sting. Some people get sick and die when they are infected with even a small amount of HIV virus, and others can remain HIV-negative and healthy even when repeatedly exposed.

In addition to genetic predisposition, all human beings—even identical twins—develop slightly different *immune systems* depending on exactly what disease-causing agents they are exposed to over the course of their lives. As a result, each person is affected by the exact same disease-causing agents in different ways.

Because of this combination of genetic predisposition and the personal history of each person's immune system, whenever a new disease comes along, some people's immune systems just happen

Life is like a tree, and its root is consciousness. Therefore, once we tend the root, the tree as a whole will be healthy. Nature controls healing from this deeper level already, for every cell participates in the body's inner intelligence, responding to the patient's thoughts, emotions, desires, beliefs, and self-image.
—DEPAK CHOPRA

to be well suited to fighting it off, while others just aren't.

Whenever a large group of people is exposed to a *virus*, many people will become infected and will be antibody-positive, while others will be able to fight off the infection itself and remain antibody-negative. Of those who do become infected, some will be affected very mildly, if at all, while others will be affected quite severely, and may even die as a result. This has been true for all viruses that humans have ever been exposed to, and is certainly also true about HIV.

In addition, there are many different strains of HIV, some of which are more dangerous than others. For example, HIV-2, which is the most common in West Africa, seems to produce less severe disease than does the HIV-1 strain that is the more common in the rest of the world. Within these strains, there may well be differences or substrains that are different. There is a great deal of current interest and research into the possibility that some rarer strains are benign and cause no symptoms. This is one reason why people who are HIV-positive need to practice safer sex even with others who are also HIV-positive, but may carry a subtly different strain of the HIV virus.

Of course, the answers to these questions are very important to discover, but on another level, it really doesn't matter to those of us that must deal with HIV/AIDS on a daily basis.

HAVING HIV DOES NOT MEAN YOU HAVE AIDS

Many people confuse HIV and AIDS. People who are infected with HIV are said to be HIV-positive or to have HIV Disease. They may appear perfectly healthy and live for years or even decades without getting AIDS, although their immune systems are often weakened over the years as the disease progresses.

AIDS is not really a single disease, but rather a

collection of many diseases that can occur only if the immune system is very badly damaged at the later stages of HIV infection.

Having AIDS means that someone meets certain very specific medical criteria defined by the Centers for Disease Control (CDC), which we will discuss later. If they meet these requirements, then they have AIDS. If they don't meet them, then they are simply "HIV-positive."

Since so many people confuse and misuse the two terms, the media has coined the term "full-blown AIDS" to emphasize when they mean CDC-defined AIDS, not just HIV-positive. This only confuses things more, because it implies that there might be "a mild case of AIDS," which is like talking about "a mild case of pregnancy."

THE SPECTRUM OF HIV DISEASE
Some people feel that the term AIDS, although precise, is not very meaningful in describing how healthy one is at any given time. Some people with AIDS remain healthy for a dozen years or more, and some people who are only HIV-positive can be seriously ill and even die before they ever become defined as having AIDS.

The future belongs to those who believe in the beauty of their dreams.

—ELEANOR ROOSEVELT

Which label one gets has very little to do with how healthy one is at any given time. Because of this, many prefer to describe HIV/AIDS as a single disease along a spectrum, which has many levels ranging from very healthy to gravely ill.

To reflect this, we will refer to it as HIV/AIDS throughout the book when we are describing the whole spectrum and use HIV to mean the virus itself, and AIDS to mean CDC-defined "full-blown AIDS."

THE PROGRESSION OF HIV/AIDS
When a person is exposed to the HIV virus, say through unsafe sex or by sharing injection drug equipment, one of two things happens.

When you go to bed
with someone, you
also go to bed with
their karma. This
may be crystal clear
when it comes to
something like AIDS
or herpes, but it's
not so obvious in
terms of more subtle
psychological stuff.
Without getting
fancy and esoteric,
I'll just say that
when you have sex
with someone, they
get their karmic
books into you.
Intentionally or
unintentionally, they
manipulate you in
terms of their needs,
their goals, their
dramas, even their
sense of propriety.
They work on your
mind and get you
involved in their
destiny. Even if you
never see them
again, they leave an
impact. So you
want to be very
careful who it is you
go to bed with. All
that glitters is
definitely not gold.
—WILLIAM
ASHOKA ROSS

Often nothing happens, and that person remains uninfected. This does not mean that they are in any way immune to getting infected with HIV in the future, it just means that they were lucky. We will discuss this more fully later in the chapter.

Unfortunately, not everyone is so lucky, and sometimes a person becomes infected with HIV. Almost as soon as they are, they are able to infect others.

When someone is exposed to any virus, the body produces tiny proteins in the blood, called antibodies, that help fight that specific virus, and only that virus. It takes the body some time to produce enough antibodies to be able to show up on the current tests. This length of time between actual infection and testing positive is called the "window period."

Almost 95% of those who are infected with HIV will have developed enough antibodies to be detectable within 6–12 weeks after infection. Almost all the remaining 5% will have developed detectable levels within 6 months. Many people incorrectly believe that HIV can somehow "hide" for years without being able to be detected. This is not true.

A "positive" HIV test result means that you have been infected with the HIV virus. A "negative" HIV test result can mean one of two things, either:

- You have NOT been infected with the HIV virus.

—OR—

- You MIGHT HAVE been infected with the HIV virus within the last six months, and it has not yet shown up on the test.

Sometimes during this window period, people may experience flulike symptoms, including fatigue, swollen glands, and night sweats as the immune system tries unsuccessfully to fight off the virus. Many people experience no symptoms at all. Since these symptoms are so general and could be caused by any number of different things, they have very little value in predicting whether someone has been infected with HIV.

For some period of time, perhaps a very long time, the body remains more or less unaffected. This phase is known as "HIV Asymptomatic" because there are no serious symptoms.

For most people, eventually the HIV virus begins very slowly to weaken the immune system. This may take months, or years, or decades to begin.

As the immune system weakens, the body may eventually not be able to fight off some diseases. Every person is different, and responds to various diseases differently, so it is difficult to say which of these symptoms are a direct result of a weak immune system, and which may be from another cause.

There has never been a really good way of directly measuring the strength of a person's immune system. One measure is to count the number of T-cells per milliliter of blood (we will discuss this shortly). Unfortunately, many other factors affect this count, and the test itself is not very accurate. Although any one reading is not very meaningful, many sets of T-cell counts taken over time do show a trend that can give some idea of how strong the immune system is.

Eventually, if enough symptoms occur, the gray area is crossed and a person is considered "HIV Symptomatic." This was once called AIDS-Related Complex, or ARC, although this term is rarely used today because of the lack of any clear definition.

A person is said to have "AIDS" once he or she has met any one of the twenty-five criteria that are listed in the CDC (Centers for Disease Control) definition of who has, and who does not have AIDS. This definition was last updated in 1993.

These opportunistic infections and other conditions include certain forms of candidiasis; cervical cancer; coccidioidomycosis; cryptococcosis; cryptosporidiosis; cytomegalovirus; encephalopathy; herpes simplex; histoplasmosis; isosporiasis; KS (Kaposi's sarcoma); lymphoma; MAI (mycobacterium avium intracellulare); mycobacterium tuberculosis; PCP (pneumocystis carinii pneumonia); pneumonia; progressive multifocal leukoencephalopathy; salmonella septicemia; TB (tuberculosis); toxoplasmosis; wasting syndrome; or a helper T4-cell count below two hundred.

HIV INFECTION IS ALMOST 100% PREVENTABLE

As viruses go, HIV is very weak. To infect a new host, the virus must swim in a fresh liquid from a person who is already HIV infected directly into another person's bloodstream. This can happen directly, through an open cut in the skin, or absorption can occur through a mucus membrane, the tissues which surround the five or six "wet openings" we have in our bodies, such as the mouth and rectum.

HIV is very choosy, and can only swim in liquids that contain special sorts of cells. The only body fluids that contain enough of these cells to enable HIV infection are human blood, semen, vaginal lubrication, and breast milk.

HIV cannot wait around outside the body for very long, because it is "anaerobic," meaning that it is destroyed almost immediately in air. It also cannot exist for very long if it becomes dried out, cooled or heated, or exposed to light.

Almost two-thirds of all adults with AIDS became infected through unsafe sexual contacts and about a quarter were infected through sharing injection drug equipment. Less than 10% were infected through all other methods combined, including mother-to-child,

Living well and beautifully and justly are all one thing.

—SOCRATES

The art of medicine consists of amusing the patient while nature cures the disease.

—VOLTAIRE

blood transfusions and other medical direct blood-to-blood contact.

About one-third of the time, a mother who is HIV-positive will pass the virus on to her baby through the umbilical cord and in her milk. The rest of the time, the baby is not infected. There is currently a great deal of research on this phenomenon.

HIV is not classified as either "contagious" or "infectious," since it can only be transmitted through direct contact. There HAS NEVER BEEN a single case of HIV transmission attributed to any method of exposure other than direct contact with infected blood, semen, vaginal lubrication, or breast milk.

In the millions of cases of HIV infection, there has never been even one case of infection through: airborne particles, coughing, dirty laundry, hugging someone with AIDS, eating food prepared by someone with AIDS, kissing, mosquitoes, public places, sharing food or eating utensils, sex (providing that each person's blood, semen, vaginal lubrication, and/or breast milk NEVER enters the other person's body), sneezing, spitting, swimming, toilets, or touching.

Scientists have conducted extensive tests looking for HIV in other body fluids, such as saliva, tears, sweat, urine, vomit, or fecal matter. Only the smallest trace amounts have ever been found. These amounts are far too small to cause infection, although any of these body fluids could also contain small amounts of blood that could carry HIV infection.

It is important to understand that the laboratory method that they use to check for HIV is one of the most accurate tests used in medicine today.

The skin is a surprisingly GOOD barrier against the HIV virus. HIV-infected body fluids on the skin WILL NOT cause infection, unless there is an open cut of some sort, that allows the liquid into the body. Many people, however, do have open cuts that they don't think about as such, for example, bleeding fin-

The great majority of us are required to live a life of constant, systematic duplicity. Your health is bound to be affected if, day after day, you say the opposite of what you feel, if you grovel before what you dislike and rejoice at what brings you nothing but misfortune. Our nervous system isn't just a fiction; it's a part of our physical body, and our soul exists in space, and is inside us, like the teeth in our mouth. It can't be forever violated with impunity.

—BORIS PASTERNAK Dr. Zhivago

gernail cuticles, paper cuts, or even freshly brushed teeth.

HIV/AIDS is an equal opportunity disease. It does not care who you are, or what you identify yourself to be. What you do with whom is what puts you at risk for HIV infection.

When someone has unsafe sex or performs any other "risky" activity, that person is being indirectly exposed to everyone his or her partner has been with for the last ten to twenty years. This means that the effective number of people that you have been indirectly exposed to grows exponentially with the number of people that you were actually exposed to.

For example, let's say you start dating at age 16, and when you are 18, you have (unprotected) sex. Since you were both virgins, you have now been exposed to one person. Then you break up, and date someone else for two years. Assuming your new partner has had an identical sexual history, when you have sex with him or her you will be exposed to THREE people, because he or she had been to bed with one other person previously $(1+1+1 = 3)$. Two years later you go to bed with someone else whose history and that of his or her partners is identical to yours. You will now have been exposed to SEVEN people, since this new partner also had three previous exposures $(3+1+3 = 7)$. At this rate, by the age of 30 you would have been exposed to 127 people. With the current rates of infection, at least one of those will probably be HIV-positive.

The reports of my death are greatly exaggerated.
—MARK TWAIN
In a cable from London to the Associated Press

If, instead, you were exposed to two people each year, all of whom had the same number of cumulative partners, in your fifteenth year of sexual activity you could have been exposed to as many as 8,589,934,591 (eight billion!) different people, assuming that no one was duplicated on more than one person's list. Of course there would have to be duplicates, since there are only five and one-half billion people on the whole planet.

Even if you went to bed with just one person in your life, that person might have been with a two-a-month-person, so that you could be exposed to thousands of people without knowing it.

WHAT IS SAFE? WHAT IS RISKY?

"Risk" means that there is some chance of danger. There is no such thing as risk-free behavior. You could be killed by a jumbo jet crashing into your home while you are reading this paragraph. The next time you go near the window, you could be shot by a stray bullet from a freak drive-by shooting. The next snack you take from the kitchen could have been tainted with poison by some psychopath at the supermarket. When you next drive in a car, you could be killed in an auto accident.

Of course, all these things could happen, but the odds are so remote that we think of them as impossible. But they are not. In fact, one person out of every 1,856,546 is killed every day as a result of an automobile accident. Most of us consider this an acceptable risk for the benefits of being able to get around by car. Many of us try to decrease the risk of being injured by owning safer cars, properly maintaining them, using safety belts, etc.

The same factors apply to sex. There is no such thing as safe sex. It might cause a heart attack, a stroke, throw your back out, or get you murdered by a jealous lover. You might also get gonorrhea, syphilis, hepatitis, herpes, or crabs. But there are things you can do to reduce the risk to the point where you can comfortably include sex in your life.

In terms of HIV, any activity that allows one person's blood, semen, vaginal lubrication, or breast milk to enter another person's body CREATES A RISK OF HIV infection. Some people like to play a game. They call some activities "very risky" and other activities "much less risky." So far, that's totally reasonable.

We have to face the fact that either all of us are going to die together or we are going to learn to live together and if we are to live together, we have to talk.
—ELEANOR ROOSEVELT

Then they make the jump that the "not so risky" things are OK to do.

Drinking poison is very risky. Pointing a six-shooter at your head and pulling the trigger with five empty chambers and one bullet in it is much less risky. This does not make Russian Roulette safe. If you play it long enough, you will lose. The same is true about sex and any other activity that has the potential to get the blood, semen, vaginal lubrication, or breast milk from a person whose HIV status you are not absolutely certain of inside your body.

Latex is one of the best barriers known against the HIV virus. EVERY TIME you engage in any "insertive sexual behavior" including oral, vaginal, or anal sex, use a fresh latex condom (rubber), dental dam, or glove and plenty of water-based lubricant. This will prohibit HIV infection so long as the barrier does not break or leak. Oil-based lubricants such as baby oil, Crisco, hand lotion, and Vaseline can increase the possibility of the condom breaking.

Sometimes condoms do break or leak anyway. This is almost always due to people failures not mechanical failures. Condoms manufactured in the USA must have a failure rate of not more than 4 out of 1,000. Many people claim a higher failure rate, but this is almost always attributable to improper usage (usually due to lack of proper training). Again, these statistics can be hotly argued, but for this example, let's use 4 out of 1,000.

One controversial study of heterosexual intercourse suggests that under "optimum circumstances," out of every 100 "episodes of unprotected sex" an HIV-positive man will infect a women one time. Of course, if the woman is near her period, or is a virgin, or any of a dozen other factors, the odds skyrocket, but for argument's sake, let's use the number 1 out of 100.

If you accept these numbers, then by simple arithmetic, under optimum circumstances, out of every

At college age, you can tell who is best at taking tests and going to school, but you can't tell who the best people are. That worries the hell out of me.

BARNABY C.
KEENEY

100,000 "episodes of unprotected sex" an HIV-positive man will infect a woman 4 times, which is equivalent to 1 out of 25,000.

Is this completely safe? Absolutely not. Is it an acceptable risk? That is an individual decision. For me it might be, and for someone else, it might not.

The important thing is to acknowledge that NOTHING is ever risk-free. Risk is a spectrum, and you must evaluate how much risk you are willing to take. Remember that "low risk" still has some risk, and some people will become infected through low-risk activities. The important thing is to change your behavior to LOWER as much as possible whatever risks you are exposed to.

I often ask audiences, if you knew your physician or surgeon had AIDS, would you switch doctors? Would you drive an extra half hour out of your way to go to a doctor you believed to be HIV-free?

The odds of being killed on the highway during that 30-mile drive are significantly higher than the odds of becoming HIV infected (which might only lead to an earlier death) from an HIV-positive health-care worker. In other words, it is much SAFER to stay with the doctor with HIV/AIDS than to drive half an hour to an HIV-free doctor.

As we have said before, it is very difficult to become HIV infected, and HIV itself is destroyed almost immediately if it becomes dried out, cooled off, or exposed to light. Nevertheless, many people like to be extra careful about any possible exchange of any blood, semen, vaginal lubrication, or breast milk. Since you never know for certain someone else's HIV status, it is probably best NEVER to share personal items such as toothbrushes, razors, and other personal or medical equipment.

Any items that do come in contact with blood, semen, vaginal lubrication, or breast milk should be disposed of properly or disinfected by soaking in

Sometimes I wonder if men and women suit each other. Perhaps they should live next door and just visit now and then.

—KATHARINE HEPBURN

bleach or rubbing alcohol and then rinsed in plenty of water. These precautions are really far more than are necessary, but it is better to be extra careful.

WHO SHOULD PRACTICE "SAFER SEX"?

In the early days of this epidemic, when HIV was fairly rare outside of very specific groups and geographic locations, it was reasonable to assume that if you knew the sexual and drug history of your partner, you would be pretty safe. This is no longer the case.

Sex is just the beginning, not the end. But if you miss the beginning, you will miss the end also.

—BHAGWAN SHREE RAJNEESH

There are millions of people who are HIV-positive in the United States, and there is no way of casually telling who they are. In some communities, the rate of infection is alarmingly high.

For a number of reasons, many people will not honestly tell you their sexual history or health status. Most people who are HIV-positive do not yet know themselves. Because of the "window period" there is no way to know for sure that someone is not infected with HIV, even with the HIV test. If they tested HIV-negative more than six months ago, and have tested HIV-negative recently, then you must ask yourself if you will bet your life on the assumption that they didn't do anything risky in the meantime.

Hope for the best, but plan for the worst. Whether you are in the bedroom, beauty salon, doctor's office, or back alley, it is important that you assume everyone is HIV-positive, and act accordingly. Ask yourself "would I do THIS activity in THIS way if I knew that they had HIV or AIDS?" If not, then you probably shouldn't do it that way.

It is important to understand that there are many different strains (types) of HIV virus. This means that even if you are HIV-positive, it is important to avoid being infected by someone else who is HIV-positive, but might have a different strain of HIV. Your body might be able to cope well with the HIV you already have, but very badly with some new form.

"SAFER" GUIDELINES

To become infected with HIV, you must get infected blood directly into your bloodstream. The more HIV-infected blood, semen, vaginal lubrication, or breast milk that you get into your body, the higher the chance of becoming HIV-infected. From a purely physical point of view, this is why the passive partner is at a somewhat higher risk for unprotected sex.

When a man reaches orgasm, he ejaculates a quantity of semen (cum). If he is infected with HIV, then contact with this semen can cause infection. If he ejaculates inside of someone, then quite a lot of this infectious material will be left behind and could cause infection for a long time, until the body decomposes it. The saliva in the mouth and digestive juices in the stomach will destroy the HIV on contact, but not all of the HIV will be contacted at once.

If, on the other hand, this man were HIV-negative, the urethra, which is the mucus membrane at the tip of his penis, could come into contact with HIV-infected blood during sex from the walls of vagina, anus, or mouth. This blood could infect him. However, it could only happen while the tip of the penis was in contact with that blood, which would only be for a very short time. Again, any saliva in the mouth will destroy the HIV it contacts.

From this description of the logistics of the situation, you would rightly assume that it is very difficult to get HIV from getting a blow job. Yet it is important to understand that the HIV virus can be transmitted to and from either partner during oral, vaginal, or anal intercourse, since there is the possibility of the exchange of blood, semen, and/or vaginal lubrication in both directions. This has long been understood with other similarly transmitted diseases such as syphilis and gonorrhea, but the common myth is that HIV is not transmitted through oral sex.

Although HIV transmission is far more likely to

> *Only the united beat of sex and heart together can create ecstasy.*
>
> —ANAÏS NIN

the person performing oral sex, I know of a man who claims to have become HIV-positive through receiving oral sex as his only possible method of infection. I believe him. In his own words, "Condoms would have been a major drag, but getting HIV is a bigger drag." It's very rare to be infected with HIV in this manner. For these people, it is of very little comfort that the odds were with them, and that for a while they lucked out on a very long shot.

Any risk is risky, whether it's oral sex or any other activity. The question comes down to how much risk you are willing to take. When injecting drugs (including steroids), do not inject them using a needle that has been used by someone else. Most injecting recreational drug users who have been active a while are HIV-positive. If you must use someone else's works, shooter, or other equipment, clean out a needle, flush it out three or four times with bleach and then flush it out three or four times with clean water. Consider another way of taking the drug, or best of all, please see "Chapter 6: Doing Healthy Stuff and Avoiding Unhealthy Stuff."

TAKING "THE TEST"

What some people call the "AIDS test" is actually a test for the presence of the body's response to the HIV virus in the blood, which is called HIV antibodies.

Deciding if, when, and how to take the HIV test involves many practical, emotional, medical, legal, political, ethical, and privacy issues. The question of HIV testing also uses its own vocabulary.

To take an HIV test, you must give your "informed consent," which has two parts: first that you cannot be tested without giving your permission in writing, and second that you made the choice to get tested in full possession of all the facts and were mentally able and mature enough to understand them.

In most cases taking this test is purely voluntary,

meaning that everyone can realistically choose to take it or not to take it. This is particularly important because, as we will discuss below, some people might not be ready to take it yet. The opposite of voluntary is mandatory, meaning that you could be required to take the test. Currently, everyone in the armed forces or requesting an immigration visa for entry into the US is REQUIRED to prove that they are HIV-negative before they are accepted.

The results of any medical test, including the HIV test, can be confidential, anonymous, or blind. With a confidential test, the sample is identified as yours and the results are recorded in your medical record. The content of your medical record is only supposed to be told to those who have a legal right to know. Unfortunately, sometimes that can be a very long list, including insurance companies, employers, etc. Sometimes others find out as well.

An anonymous test is one where the sample is assigned a number, and only you know the results, hence they could not be recorded in your medical record. In a blind test, the samples are taken from many people, but they are not labeled from whom they came. No one person would know as a result of a blind test if he or she were HIV-positive, but one would know what percentage of the whole group was infected.

"Disclosure" means whom you need to tell. When HIV/AIDS was relatively rare, some states passed laws that required people who tested HIV-positive to notify everyone whom they may have infected. This is similar to how public health officials have dealt with sexually transmitted diseases such as syphilis and gonorrhea. Unfortunately, now that HIV is so widespread, contact tracing is no longer a reliable solution. Anyone who has engaged in activity that is considered risky for HIV infection should consider taking the antibody test. As mentioned earlier, everyone should act as if

No one can make you feel inferior without your consent.

—ELEANOR ROOSEVELT

the other person were HIV infected anyway.

A few years ago, most people chose NOT to get tested because finding out had very few practical benefits, as there were no treatments available, and there was a considerable risk of discrimination. The advice was to act as if you were HIV-positive regardless of your status.

The life which is unexamined is not worth living.
—SOCRATES

THIS IS NO LONGER THE BEST ADVICE. Today, there are many treatments and other actions that you can take to slow the progression of HIV Disease, and there are much better privacy and antidiscrimination laws for people with HIV/AIDS.

In most cases, if you are having an HIV test, there must be some possibility, no matter how remote, that it could come back positive. If there wasn't at least a remote possibility, you wouldn't be taking the test. Since there is a possibility that the test will prove you are infected with HIV, it is important that you have the information and other resources necessary to cope with that possibility. If you do not, you might choose to postpone taking the test until you can "clear the decks" emotionally.

Taking the HIV test is a very frightening process for most people. It's important to get proper counseling *both before and after testing*. Being told that you are HIV-positive is never easy to take, but some people may not be emotionally prepared to learn of a positive test result. These people should probably wait a few months and perhaps seek professional counseling. For example, people who are newly clean and sober, newly in or out of a relationship or job, or anyone who has recently undergone a major life change might consider waiting a bit until things settle down.

THE WELLNESS SPECTRUM

Here in America, we believe that being healthy and being ill are two separate, distinct states. If you are sick, you need to go to a doctor to be made well, and if you are well, you might want to diet and exercise to be more attractive. In reality, "wellness" is really more of a spectrum, a gray scale of levels of health.

"Western" medicine focuses on the treatment and cure of disease, which is very different from the "Eastern" perspective of enhancing health and longevity. Today, we're starting to realize what our friends in Japan, China, and the rest of the "East" have known for thousands of years: when it comes to health, it is much easier to keep a body healthy than it is to heal it once it's broken, diseased, run-down or ill. What's more, the body itself is the most remarkable physician there is, and given a little encouragement, it can heal itself far better than human doctors can. The most important person in the healing process is the person who's doing the healing—the patient, not the doctor.

We call this view "Holistic Medicine," meaning that it deals with the whole person, not treating health as if it were separate from the rest of that person's life. Neither does it approach illness as if sickness and health were black and white. Of course they're not. Health is a spectrum, and sickness is purely a point on that spectrum.

Most of us learned as kids that there are two things you can be, and they are "healthy" or "sick." If you're sick, you get to stay home from school, and if you're really sick, you go to a doctor, who will do something or give you something that will make you healthy again.

In the grown-up world, though, things aren't so simple. There is no such thing as being healthy or sick. These terms simply describe positions along a spectrum of "WELLNESS." Regardless of how healthy you might be, you could always get a little healthier.

You can learn to follow the inner self, the inner physician that tells you where to go. Healing is simply attempting to do more of those things that bring joy and fewer of those things that bring pain.

—O. CARL SIMONTON

HOW THE IMMUNE SYSTEM WORKS
Every living thing is able to fight off most diseases and repair itself. That is how we stay alive. The immune system is that part of our bodies that fights off diseases

and heals injuries. For example, when you get a cold (which is, by the way, also caused by an "incurable" virus), your own body's immune system creates antibodies in the blood that help fight off that particular disease. Taking aspirin, or any other medicine, does not help cure the cold, it only makes the symptoms less visible while the body "cures" itself.

Some people inherit weakened (deficient) immune systems from their parents, others may develop them as a result of extreme age or serious illness, but people with HIV/AIDS got (acquired) their immune deficiency as a result of becoming infected with the HIV virus.

Human blood is made up of many parts. The red blood cells carry oxygen to all the cells throughout the body. They are also what gives blood its color. The white blood cells fight disease. There are many different types of white blood cells. Some of these are called the T4 helper cells. Other names for these same cells are CD4 cells or T4 cells. No one is exactly sure what they do, or how they do it, but they seem to help fight disease. Normal, healthy people seem usually to have about 800 to 1,200 of them in each milliliter (about 1/5 teaspoon) of blood. People with weakened immune systems often have only 400 to 700 per milliliter, and people with AIDS sometimes have fewer than 200. There are some people who have only a few T4 helper cells per milliliter, yet continue to be healthy.

Many factors affect a person's T-cell count, and it can change greatly from day to day. In addition, the test itself is not very accurate, and may be off by 20% or more each time. As a result, T-cell counts only give a very general idea of how weak or strong a person's immune system is. Unfortunately, this is a very common test, and many people mistakenly believe that it is an accurate indication of how well or sick they are.

The way people talk about viruses, one would

think that they are little animals. They are not. In fact, they are not even considered to be technically "alive" because they are not able to reproduce by themselves. A virus is a special type of cell. It attaches itself to a living cell inside the body and uses that host cell's reproductive system to make copies of itself.

Anytime a virus gets inside your body, the immune system creates antibodies, which are another special type of blood cell, designed to attack that specific virus and help the body destroy it. Antibodies to one virus will not attack any other virus. Once your body has antibodies to a specific virus, those antibodies will remain in your blood for the rest of your life. Sometimes, those antibodies will prevent you from getting that virus again, such as what happens with chicken pox.

WOMEN, CHILDREN, AND HIV

Most of the information about people with HIV/AIDS refers to men who are aged 25 to 50, because they make up 75% of all CDC-documented cases of AIDS. So far in the US women account for only 11%, and children and adolescents for a mere 2%. Unfortunately, these are also the fastest growing groups of all people with HIV/AIDS.

Statistically, women die twice as fast after being diagnosed with AIDS as do men. This is because they are generally diagnosed very late in their condition. Often women (and their gynecologists) ignore chronic infections for months and years. Women are excluded from many clinical drug trials because of the liability of possible pregnancy and supposed hormonal complications. Lastly, women as a group—particularly poorer women—tend to have less access to health care than do men because of family responsibilities.

Many people find it surprising to learn that pregnant women who are infected with HIV do not necessarily infect their unborn child. HIV is only

In Germany they came first for the Communists, and I didn't speak up because I wasn't a Communist. Then they came for the Jews, and I didn't speak up because I wasn't a Jew. Then they came for the trade unionists, and I didn't speak up because I wasn't a trade unionist. Then they came for the Catholics, and I didn't speak up because I was a Protestant. Then they came for me— and by that time no one was left to speak up.
—PASTOR MARTIN NIEMOELLER

Living Positively in a World with HIV/AIDS 99

transmitted by blood, semen, vaginal lubrication, or breast milk, NONE of which are necessarily shared with the fetus. Many people mistakenly believe that the mother's blood somehow goes into the fetus. It does not. The fetus is a separate, living entity with its own separate blood supply that absorbs oxygen and other nutrients through the placenta wall.

All babies do, however, get a complete set of the mother's antibodies at birth. If the mother is HIV antibody-positive, then the baby will also have the HIV antibodies, however, ONLY about 10–35% of those babies will actually have the HIV virus. Perhaps as many as two-thirds of babies who are not breast-fed by HIV-positive mothers will revert to being HIV-negative within 6–18 months after birth.

It is interesting to know that while a man's ejaculatory liquid, semen (cum), may be HIV-infected, the actual sperm cannot be. Although current medical technology is not able to separate viable sperm from the semen, someday it may well be able to do so. If that happens, then HIV-positive men may be able to father children without risk of HIV infection.

To know that you do not know is the best. To pretend to know when you do not know is disease.
—LAO-TZU

CHAPTER 8

TAKING CHARGE OF YOUR OWN HEALTH CARE

> **6** Take an active role in your health care. Letting even the best health-care professional choose your treatment is like letting a travel agent choose where you're going on vacation. Both can have invaluable input, knowledge, and experience, but they can't know what's right for you unless you ask questions, do your homework, learn all you can, evaluate your options, and communicate how you feel.
>
> Sometimes these folks forget that their main job is to advise you, coach you, and provide you with the information you need to make your own choices and take your own actions. "Reeducate" those who want to dictate "what you have to do." You don't have to do anything. There are no magic answers in life that are right for all people at all times.
>
> Seek out people who will listen to you, respect you, and work with you as a member of your team. Work in collaboration with them, but don't let them bully you into doing anything that you really don't believe in. Remember that it is your body; you make the final decisions; you have the right to keep asking "why?" and the right to say "no" to anything that you don't fully understand and agree with.

FINDING OUT IF YOU ARE HIV-POSITIVE

Whatever path you follow to treat HIV/AIDS, you must first know if you are HIV-positive, what the current state of your immune system is, and be informed as to your choices. If you don't have the necessary information, then all that you can do is hide. And, unfortunately, hiding doesn't work very well at all against the HIV virus. As Sir Francis Bacon wrote almost four hundred years ago, "Knowledge is power."

I cannot stress this enough: HIV/AIDS can be a treatable, chronic condition that you can learn to live with, *but only if you know about it.* Finding out for the first time that you are HIV-positive when you are being admitted to the emergency room with an AIDS-related condition makes everything so much more difficult.

Almost everyone feels a little uncomfortable talking about sexuality and drug use. As a result, a lot of people cover up facts, or just plain lie. You have to assume everyone you've come in contact with is HIV-positive, so if there is even the most remote chance that you may have been exposed to the HIV virus, it's probably a good idea to get tested either once a year or six months after your last possible exposure.

If you don't know for sure, get tested for HIV every year, or as needed. If you are HIV-positive, get a complete physical with blood work at least twice a year, if not more often.

HIV TESTING OPTIONS

There are many different options for getting tested. They are all very simple, although emotionally they can be very difficult. Which one you choose depends on your personal needs:

◆ An important new option is the at-home HIV test. Pending final FDA approval—which hopefully will have been received by the time you read this—you will be able to purchase a mail-in HIV testing kit at your local pharmacy. Results take about a week. Mail-in HIV testing offers the most privacy, as each test kit has a unique ID number but not the person's name. Telephone counseling is available by calling an 800 number, and although this isn't as good as a sit-down visit with a wonderful doctor, it is far better than the complete lack of counseling that 85 percent who are tested today must face.

- Go to a private clinic. Medical records may be kept and it can cost $100 or more, but you can probably get negative results in 15 minutes. Positive results take a few days, and counseling is sometimes not as good as it could be. At many places you can pay cash and use a made-up name so no records are kept.

- A public clinic is usually anonymous and free or at very low cost, but may have a many-week wait to get an appointment and may take two weeks to get results and counseling.

Be extremely careful about ever taking an HIV test where the results will go on your permanent record, such as with your insurance company, employer, or even your doctor's office. It's probably a good idea to take an anonymous test first, since the surprise of an unexpected positive test "on the record" has the *possibility* of costing you your job, your insurance, and causing other complications. All this can be avoided with careful planning.

For more information, refer to "Chapter 7: Becoming Your Own Medical Expert" and the section on the HIV antibody test.

I believe that anyone can conquer fear by doing the things he fears to do, provided he keeps doing them until he gets a record of successful experiences behind him.

—ELEANOR ROOSEVELT

THE SHORTCOMINGS OF THE WESTERN MEDICAL VIEWPOINT

I'm a great fan of "Western" doctors, and I'm very glad to be living in a part of the world where medical technology is so advanced. The miracle of modern "Western" medicine does, however, have its down side: it tends to treat symptoms well, but is less successful with the underlying causes.

"Western" medicine is very scientific, but this often makes it seem cold and impersonal, treating sick bodies like machines to be fixed by increasingly clever technology. This is too bad, because symptoms are the only way the body has to tell you that something is out of balance and needs to be taken care of before it does more damage.

All of us are partly to blame. We have come to demand and depend on quick fixes from our doctors: "magic bullet" drugs and miracle surgeries that remove the symptoms without any effort on our part. Rather than seeing our doctors as "health coaches" to help us keep ourselves well, most people only turn to a doctor as a last resort, often when it's too late, and we are seriously ill. Repairs are always more costly and more risky than prevention.

With the exception of "sports medicine" and a few other new fields of study, "Western" medicine focuses on illness rather than on health. Doctors study how to make sick people well rather than studying why healthy people don't get sick in the first place. The old adage "an ounce of prevention is better than a pound of cure" hasn't reached widespread application in our society just yet.

It wasn't always this way. Over twenty-four hundred years ago, the father of modern medicine, Hippocrates, wrote that "prayer indeed is good, but while calling on the gods, each person should lend a hand themselves."

It wasn't until the mid-1800s, when Louis Pasteur and others discovered that germs could cause disease, that these ideas started to get lost. Today, traditional "Western" medical schools teach that "cases" are somehow not people, but broken mechanical, biological, and chemical machines that need fixing. In Western medicine, healing is not thought to be significantly affected by psychological, emotional, or spiritual factors.

Doctors are viewed as master mechanics whose skill in performing the diagnosis and treatment somehow caused the healing. Patients are merely treated as passive receptacles who, like ignorant children, cannot possibly understand the complexities of the situation, and are best seen but not heard. Certainly patients are often made to feel they have no business meddling in medical matters.

Unfortunately, disease, healing, and the body simply don't work that way. The body has a profound ability to heal itself. Doctors are merely the coaches and medical consultants to the patients. Many doctors still don't understand this. Perhaps one of the reasons that doctors, as a group, have one of the highest suicide rates in our society is because they mistakenly believe that illness and death are somehow failures on their part, and that if only they had done more, or known more, the patient could have been fine.

WHO DOES THE HEALING?
When you have been sick in the past, who "made you well again?" Depending on your age, most of you probably answered your mother, your spouse, or some health professional. Although these people certainly may have helped, your own body healed itself. Sure, it might have *needed* a little help, but your body did almost all the work.

Imagine going into a travel agent and waiting hours to see a "travel expert." After being asked a few questions—without really any conversation—you are

> We have not lost faith, but we have transferred it from God to the medical profession.
> —GEORGE BERNARD SHAW

> You may fool all the people some of the time; you can even fool some of the people all of the time; but you can't fool all of the people all of the time.
> —ABRAHAM LINCOLN

handed your tickets, and told what dates you will be taking your vacation, where you will be going, what you will be doing, and how much you have been billed.

If you protest, you will be told in a firm voice that you couldn't possibly know all the millions of details involved and that you should trust the experts. If you complain further, you will be considered "a nut" in need of counseling.

Millions of us have a very similar experience when we try to deal with the modern health-care industry. Doctors are viewed as infallible experts and patients as stupid little children who don't know what's best for them.

No medical "expert" can ever understand your exact situation better than you can. What is more important, if you take the time to do your homework, ask loads of questions, and really listen, you—not your doctor—are the best person to make the medical decisions. This is what the Nobel Prize–winning doctor Albert Schweitzer called "listening to the healer within us all."

TREATMENT COCKTAILS

If a man does not keep pace with his companions, perhaps it is because he hears a different drummer. Let him step to the music which he hears, however measured or far away.

—HENRY DAVID THOREAU

As I keep pointing out, because HIV/AIDS is so complex, there are no simple answers or no single treatment that works for everybody all the time. Everyone is different, and their needs change over time.

Most people end up doing a number of different things together. Each person has to find what combination of things work for him or her: which medications, drugs, supplements, daily activities, treatments, and other actions that they "mix together" into what is often called their own personal "treatment cocktail."

Although some feel that traditional "Western" medical treatments alone are the right choice, most people find it best to supplement these with a variety of alternative, holistic, or "Eastern" medical practices, as well as some sort of psychotherapy, support group, spiritual or inspirational path.

Bernie Siegel, the noted surgeon who helps "exceptional" cancer patients flourish, "encourages you to use all of your assets—yourself, the medical profession and your spiritual faith."

Every year there are more and better "ingredients" and "recipes" for the "treatment cocktail" that help more people stay healthier longer. Hopefully, this book will help point you in some new directions and suggest some new possibilities for you to try as you seek to discover the path that works best for you right now.

OLD WIVES' TALES, FOLK REMEDIES, AND HOLISTIC MEDICINE

Nowadays, we tend to look at traditional Western doctors working in traditional Western hospitals as the only source of reliable, useful medical assistance. For some reason we believe that medical treatment is separate from the rest of our life, and that the people who perform this treatment on us are somehow special.

Who is a "health-care professional?" To most of us, this is synonymous with "physician" but it need not be. It may be an allopath, chiropractor, dentist, dietitian, gynecologist, homeopath, massage therapist, medical consultant or advisor, medical technician, midwife, naturopath, nurse, nutritionist, obstetrician, optometrist, osteopath, paramedic, pediatrician, physical therapist, surgeon, therapist, or one of hundreds of other medical specialists. If it's a mental or emotional problem, we might think of psychiatrist, psychologist, social worker, therapist, and counselor.

And these are just some of the names we use in our society. In other cultures, you might seek out the local barber, fortune teller, medicine man (or woman),

The greatest revolution in our generation is the discovery that human beings, by changing the inner attitudes of their minds, can change the outer aspects of their lives.
—WILLIAM JAMES

faith healer, shaman, witch doctor, hypnotist, herbalist, acupuncturist, or tribal elder.

In some other parts of the world, less of a distinction is made between a person's physical, mental, and spiritual health, so one might consult with a priest, minister, rabbi, mullah, pundit, lama, guru, or other spiritual advisor.

Any sufficiently advanced technology is indistinguishable from magic.
    —ARTHUR C. CLARKE

Every culture since the beginning of human history has sought ways of helping the sick. Every culture and every generation has its unique form of folk medicine. It's important not to dismiss these.

After all, our "high-tech" medical treatments were all discovered either by trial and error or by studying what worked in folk medicine. Almost every "Western" drug is really just some naturally occurring substance that has been refined and purified from a plant, mineral, or animal.

Even the best "Western" scientific minds are sometimes a little prejudiced against other cultures and traditions. Too often they believe that if they see something but don't have a theory that can explain it, then it can't be real.

This is nonsense. We ask advanced people all over the world to accept that our "Western" medicines are superior to *all* of their folk medicines. Why can't we accept that *perhaps some of these* folk medicines and practices might be superior to ours?

I remember a time when chiropractors were considered nonmedical quacks and when acupuncture was thought to be a useless, pagan ritual. Now both are commonly accepted as an effective means of treatment. Despite the success of "Western" medicine, there are so many problems it simply doesn't address very well, problems routinely treated with wonderful results by other methods.

Since "Western" medicine doesn't have all the answers for HIV/AIDS, it's a good idea to look at some other healing traditions and resources. It's foolish not to shop around. Just because we don't understand how a drug or treatment works doesn't mean it can't be effective.

On the other hand, just because something is widely accepted or has a sound theory behind it, doesn't mean it really works, or that it will work for you. Only the test of time and careful scientific study can prove that.

EXPERTS, CHARLATANS, CON MEN, AND QUACKS

In my office there is a very impressive bronze plaque mounted on walnut that proclaims:

Mark de Solla Price
Certified Expert

Always listen to experts. They'll tell you what can't be done and why. Then do it.

—ROBERT HEINLEIN

As I said, very impressive. It means a lot to me, and it took a long time to get it. Six to eight weeks to be exact. And it cost $49 plus shipping and handling.

Of course, it's only meant as a joke, but it does help remind me of three very important facts:

1. It pays to be a little cynical and question appearances.
2. Having an impressive title, or rock-solid credentials, or being recognized as an expert doesn't necessarily mean you have all the right answers.
3. When it comes to something as complex as HIV/AIDS, there is no such thing as an expert, because no one can know all the right answers for everyone.

Seriously, though, some of the best minds in medicine are working on HIV/AIDS, and many people have amassed a lot of important knowledge and skill.

There are also a lot of well-meaning fools, opportun-istic con men, profiteering "businessmen," and quack doctors. The trouble is, how do you tell who is who?

CERTIFIED EXPERTS

In America anyone can grow up to be The President. The joke goes, if you look at the last few holders of the office, you can see it's true: *anyone can be president*, regardless of his qualifications, experience, or abilities.

In this country, to legally drive an automobile, one must meet specific requirements, pass a standardized test, and continue to comply with certain rules. Surprisingly, very few professionals have to go through such a formal process.

Authority, you tell us that we're no good. Well, authority, you're no good.
—ANONYMOUS

Over the years, I've made a pretty good living as a consultant and motivational speaker. What credentials do I have for doing this? Although I do have all sorts of training, certifications, and professional memberships, when it comes right down to it I'm qualified to be a consultant and motivational speaker because *I say that I am qualified*. To my knowledge there is no "American Consultant and Motivational Speakers' Organization" nor are there any laws that state that it is illegal to consult or speak to others without belonging to such a group. If I'm wrong about this, please let me know.

Let's say that instead of looking to hire a doctor you need to have some other service performed—anything from repairing your car to resoling your shoes—how would you pick the right professional to do the job? Often it is difficult to know who is *professional* and who is not, until it's too late.

To help consumers know whom they can trust, people have formed trade guilds, unions, and professional organizations for hundreds of years. In some countries and in some industries, these organizations are regulated under governmental authority, but in the

United States, most are not regulated or controlled in any way.

Some of the more powerful trade organizations have even lobbied to get laws in place that make it illegal to operate without membership. Many of these organizations are reputable, others are merely public relations and marketing scams.

The problem with regulation by one's peers is that sometimes the majority is wrong. They may see something as dangerous for the customer, when it is really only dangerous to their businesses and income. Other times regulations are well-meaning, but years behind the times.

Does that mean that certifications are meaning-less? No, but it's important to consider who did the certifying.

Lastly, you might check to see who's licensed, certified, or approved by an association, trade union, or other organization that you respect. Just because they are licensed, certified, or approved, doesn't mean that they are any good. There may be far more qual-ified people who, for some reason, are not recognized by or members of this organization.

Caveat emptor is Latin for "let the buyer beware," meaning you alone are responsible for making a bad purchase. It's your choice to be a smart consumer of health-care services.

An educated consumer is our best customer.
—SY SIMS
Discount Clothing
Legend

A CHECKLIST FOR CHOOSING HEALTH-CARE PROFESSIONALS

One of the most important decisions you need to make when learning to live with any medical problem is picking the best health-care team you can. Naturally, your personal finances and the terms of your insurance or lack of insurance greatly affect your options. What-ever the situation, it's up to you to set the ground rules.

Assembling the right professionals for your own

personal health-care team is not easy. First and foremost, they must be people you trust and can talk with. They have to have the right combinations of skills, knowledge, personality, and accessibility. They need to be affordable and they need to have the time to see you. Many people don't get to choose from many options because of limited health-care benefits. It's very easy to stop your search with the first doctor or other professional you see. Don't!

It can take quite a bit of effort to find the right match even at the best of times. Trying to find someone when you are physically not at your best can be even more difficult. I cannot stress enough that regardless of your financial resources or current level of health, do not waste any time in putting together the best team that you can.

Listen to what they don't say, as well as what they do say. Those that give you a hard time about being "interviewed" for the job are probably the same people who would later on give you a hard time about letting you control your own health-care decisions.

Here's a checklist to help you choose the right people:

Skills, Qualifications, and Certifications

- Which of the hundreds of titles, philosophies, methods, and specialties does this professional identify him- or herself as belonging or subscribing to? For example, is this person a doctor of general medicine, HIV/AIDS specialist, therapeutic massage therapist, nutritionist, herbalist, aerobics instructor, or metaphysical counselor?

- How long has he or she "been in business" (practicing in this field)? How many people has he or she served? How many are currently active?

- What experience does he or she have in serving people who have needs similar to yours?

- Where did this person receive his or her training or apprenticeship? Have you heard of these schools? Is there evidence to support these claims? What about more recent "update" and "refresher" training? Is any of this HIV/AIDS-specific?

- What are his or her credentials in this field? What degrees and certifications has he or she received?

- What professional societies or "boards" does he or she belong to, and what hospitals, universities, and other organizations is he or she affiliated with? Does this person teach other professionals in this specialty?

- Who recommended this professional to you? What were that person's firsthand experiences?

- Ask around at support groups and other HIV/AIDS community resources. What experiences have others had with this sort of professional? Any general recommendations or warnings? Does anyone know about this professional firsthand?

- Does the local HIV/AIDS service organization have a referral list for this sort of professional? Is this person on that list? If not, why not?

- Do some background checking. Where might someone who has had a bad experience go to complain? Check to see if

Procrastination is the fear of success. People procrastinate because they are afraid of the success that they know will result if they move ahead now. Because success is heavy, carries a responsibility with it, it is much easier to procrastinate and live on the "someday I'll" philosophy.
—DENIS WAITLEY

there have been any complaints about this person.

- Don't be embarrassed to check personal references. Can this professional provide you with letters of recommendation or names and phone numbers of other people who have recently used his or her services?

- Does he or she sell things such as nutritional supplements, book, tapes, special tests or equipment, or training classes? Does this cause a conflict of interest? Does he or she necessarily recommend what is best for you, or whatever will make the most money? Are there other products or vendors you can work with and still use this person's services?

- Has he or she written books or conducted seminars, classes, or workshops that are geared to people like you? How much do these items or services cost?

- At which hospitals or treatment centers does this person have admitting privileges? Which are his or her preferences and why?

- What is the scope of this professional's expertise and legal authority? Is he or she able to write prescriptions or perform the procedures and other services that you may require?

- What other sorts of health-care professionals would this person encourage you to work with? Does he or she have any specific referrals?

- Does he or she give you the time you need, or do you feel rushed?

- Is he or she good at listening to you, addressing your concerns, and asking what you want, or is this person mainly talking "at you" and telling you what he or she is going to do?

- Do you feel at ease asking questions? Can he or she explain things in ways you understand? Is he or she happy to explain terms, phrases, and concepts that may be confusing to you?

- Is this person open to working with other "members of your health-care team"?— even professionals from nontraditional fields?

- Is he or she willing to take "no" for an answer if you feel strongly about something, or would you have to stop being treated by this professional?

- Will you always be seen by the same person?

- Do you feel comfortable with the whole office staff?

- Do you feel comfortable honestly discussing your private concerns and very personal subjects such as the specific details of your sexual practices, alcohol and drug use, and any other embarrassing topic if necessary?

- Is everyone on the staff comfortable working with someone dealing with HIV/AIDS?

- Would you prefer a professional that you could more closely relate to because he or she belongs to the same gender, sexual preference, age group, ethnic, cultural, religious, political, or social groups that you do, or because he or she had gone through similar experiences to what you are going through? Could you feel comfortable with the right person who did *not* meet these criteria?

- What sort of records will be kept? Who will have access to them? What diagnosis will be given? Who will this be reported to? Would you prefer any of this to be handled in a different manner? Will this professional comply?

- Does he or she focus on your personal case, or do you feel you are getting a "canned" answer?

- Are most solutions based on medications and surgeries alone, or do they include some form of behavior modification as well?

- Does this provider explain the potential benefits, risks, and costs of tests, procedures, medications, and other actions?

- Does he or she make a point of suggesting less-risky or less-costly alternatives?

Fees, Rates, Payment Policies, and Financial Affordability

- What are his or her rates? How much will a typical office visit cost? What about some standard tests and office procedures? How much will this cost per month or year? Can you afford this?

- Is there a fee for consultations over the telephone?

- How much will medications, tests, equipment, and supplies cost in addition to these fees for a typical month or year? Can you afford this?

- How much will it cost to begin, including all examinations, tests, equipment, supplies, and what have you? Can you afford this?

- What (if anything) is covered by your insurance company, health maintenance organization (HMO), or preferred provider organization (PPO)? Would you be better covered if you went elsewhere or "adjusted" how you filled out the paperwork?

- Does this provider submit claims directly to your insurance company? Will you be responsible for what is not covered?

- Is payment in full expected from you at each visit, or can you set up a payment plan or flat monthly fee? What happens if you are short of cash one month?

- Do you feel comfortable discussing your financial needs and limitations? Would you feel at ease asking how much a recommended medication or treatment might cost, and speaking up if you could not afford to do this right now?

- Does this provider accept Medicare or Medicaid?

- Do you qualify for some reduced rate, free service, outside subsidy, or assistance because of your financial needs? What do you have to do to get these benefits?

Office Practices and Appointment Scheduling

- Write down the professional's complete name, address, and phone number. Is there an alternate phone number in case of emergency? It can be useful also to know the fax machine number to be able to have information sent to the provider in a hurry.

+ Does he or she "accept" new patients or clients?

+ Is the office easy enough for you to get to, even on busy days or when you're not feeling your best?

+ What are the office hours? Do these days and times work with your life-style? What happens if you have an urgent problem at some other time?

+ How long in advance must you schedule appointments?

+ How are emergencies handled?

+ Who covers for the professional when he or she is unavailable?

+ How long does he or she allow for an average office visit? Are these "double booked"?

+ Does the practice keep on schedule, or does it often "run late"? How long, in general, might you expect to wait?

COLLABORATING WITH YOUR HEALTH-CARE TEAM

Once you have "hired on" the best health-care team that you can, you must do your part and make the best use of these great folks.

The most important thing you can do is to *listen to what they have to say.* You don't have to agree with them. You don't have to blindly do what they say. But you chose to see them, and if you are going to spend the time, money, and effort to see them, then you had better be honest with them in what you are doing and really pay attention to what they have to tell you.

From my own experience, I know that this is not easy. Often you are not at your best, either physically or mentally. Sometimes you can get disoriented by unpleasant news. Even at the best of times, you usually don't get a very long time to talk. Try some different methods to help you listen better during your appointment. Make sure that you understand all instructions and explanations. Here are a few ideas:

- Bring someone with you and have that person with you while you are talking with your health-care professional. Two sets of ears and two memories are better than one. After you leave the office review with this person exactly what was said. This way you can avoid misunderstandings.

- Bring a small tape recorder with you and record your conversation and listen to it again when you get home.

- Take careful written notes as if there was going to be a quiz on what exactly was said. For many people, the act of writing things down forces them to figure out what they don't understand.

- At the end of the conversation, repeat all the key points back to your health-care professional, for example "Just so I know I have this right, the test came back and showed . . . so you don't suggest that I . . . but you would like me to . . ." Make sure to ask "Did I get all the right information? Is there anything I forgot?"

- Specifically repeat and review the purpose of all tests, medications, and other recommendations (also see separate checklist regarding medications).

- In your HIV notebook, set aside a page to write down questions as you think of them that you would like to ask the next time you see each of your health-care professionals. Also make a note of unusual symptoms and side effects so that you can report them carefully.

- Remember to take this notebook with you to your next appointment. Make a clean copy of the questions and other items you want to cover in your appointment while you are waiting for your appointment. Review and check off this list with your health-care professional.

- Keep your own mini "chart" of key test results over time. Get a photocopy of each test report. Prepare a blood work chart or table showing you the date of each test, white blood count, platelets, T4 helper cells, T8 suppressor cells, ratio of T4/T8, percentage of T4 helper cells to total lymphocytes. This will help you spot trends that others might miss.

- If, after you have left the office, there is something that you are unclear about, don't be shy about telephoning and asking specific questions. Be reasonable about this, though. Save new questions for your next visit.

Some health-care professionals really like this technique because it shows that you value what they have to say. Others really hate it and may even refuse to work with you under these circumstances. This could be because they are (justifiably) afraid of a malpractice lawsuit, or just that it will change the doctor-patient dynamic. Frankly, if that dynamic doesn't empower and include collaborating with the patient, then it needs some changing. If he or she doesn't want to work with you this way, then you would probably be better off with a health-care professional who is more open to working in *collaboration* with you.

THE SCIENTIFIC METHOD

Now that you're working in collaboration with some of the best available HIV/AIDS experts on a very interesting case (you), you might want to follow some of the methods that scientists and doctors use to study such things.

"The Scientific Method" is a fancy way of saying that scientists observe or measure something, come up with an explanation of how it works, and do something to "prove" that it really works that way. In other words they recognize and formulate a problem, collect data through observation and experiment, and test a hypothesis or theory.

For example, using the scientific method, you might observe that you sometimes have gas in the morning. You theorize that this is from taking a pill with orange juice. You test this by taking that same pill with apple juice and again with milk without getting gas; next you drink orange juice in the morning on an empty stomach, and again no gas. Lastly, you once again take the pill with orange juice, and the gas returns.

The key is observing carefully and looking to spot trends. Realize that just because one event happens after another doesn't mean that the first caused the second. Look beyond the obvious. Sometimes it's not the pill but some other very minor factor that's causing the problem.

The last step is also very important: proving your theory by doing something that you expect to have a

Discovering the ways in which you are exceptional, the particular path you are meant to follow, is your business on this earth, whether you are afflicted or not. It's just that the search takes on a special urgency when you realize that you are mortal.
—*BERNIE SIEGEL*

particular outcome, whether it makes you feel better or not so good. This can be important, but needs to be done with care. You don't want to prove that something is fatal! Without that last step, however, you might end up avoiding a whole bunch of stuff that actually has no ill effects.

Of course, you are only one person. Doctors would call your information "anecdotal," meaning that it may be observed, but is not "proven" using a sufficiently large, statistically meaningful group.

Remember, your goal is to be healthy, not really to test out what works. If you find a treatment that works, it's foolish to stop just to "prove" that it was working for you. Another problem is determining cause and effect.

A CHECKLIST BEFORE TAKING ANY MEDICATIONS, DRUGS, OR SUPPLEMENTS

- What is it called? How do you spell that? Who are the manufacturers? Are there any other common names of this?

- Is this a brand name or a generic name? Are there some brands, sources, types, qualities, or sizes that are better than others?

- Where would you get it? Is it a prescription drug, a medication that you would buy over-the-counter at a pharmacy, a food supplement that you might get at a health food store, or an alternative treatment that you might have to get from special sources?

- Why is it being prescribed or recommended? What exactly is it supposed to do? What symptoms is it supposed to relieve, or what medical conditions is it supposed to cure or lessen?

- Has *this form* of medication or supplement been scientifically proven to be effective? Look carefully. For example, sodium (as in salt) has been proven to be the basis of all brain and neurological activity. Eating more salt, unfortunately doesn't make you any smarter.

- How quickly might you expect to see results?

- What are the potential short- and long-term risks of this treatment? How often do other people experience these problems? Have you had any bad reactions to anything similar in the past?

- Is it really necessary? What would happen if you didn't take it? Is there something that is less costly or a less-risky choice that would do as well?

- If this doesn't work well, what alternatives are there? What did people use before this was available? Remember, health-care professionals tend to use the new and fashionable treatments and forget the old ones.

- How expensive is it? Is this covered by your insurance or other health-care program? Can you afford to get this?

- Are there any programs that can provide this for free or at a reduced cost?

- Can you get any written information about this? Is it written so that you can understand it? Does the information come from a credible source or it is just advertising material from the manufacturer?

How long has it been on the market?

- What dose should you take each time? Are there any factors that might mean you should take more or less than other people, such as other medical conditions, your size/weight/age, history of drug use, current cigarette smoking, current use of alcohol and other drugs.

- How often should you take it? At what times? For example, does "every four hours" mean you have to wake up in the middle of the night to take this? For how many days? Should you keep taking it even if you feel better? What if you feel worse or experience side effects?

- Should you start out at a lower dosage and build up, start out high and taper off, or keep taking the same amount? If you need to stop, should you stop right away or slowly taper off?

- What happens if you miss a dose? Should you take it as soon as you remember? Double up next time? Skip it all together?

- If you are taking many pills each day, you might consider buying a pill-organizer with four or more compartments for each day of the week. It's easy to see if you have taken the right pills.

- Have you ever had allergic reactions or side effects to *any* drugs or foods? This might affect the choice of medications, drugs, supplements, or the dosage or follow-up procedures.

- If you do experience any side effects, write down the specific details so you can report them. It's easy to forget, and anything you notice may be important.

* What other medications, drugs, supplements are you taking? Be complete. Don't forget birth control pills, recreational drugs, alcohol, tobacco, caffeine, etc. Do you follow some special diet or nutritional program? Might any of these affect this new one?

* Are there any activities, other foods, other medications, or substances such as orange juice, alcohol, or cigarettes that you should particularly *avoid* when taking this?

* Are there any activities, foods or circumstances that make taking this easier or *more effective*?

* Ask around at support groups and local AIDS services organizations about other people's experiences. Often these folks have helpful hints about techniques or dosages for improving effectiveness, or reducing side effects. Discuss these with your health-care professional.

* When should you follow up to see if this medication, drug, or supplement is working correctly?

* Keep an *up-to-date written list* of the names and dosages of all your medications, drugs, and supplements that you are taking on a card and keep this with you in your wallet or purse. In case of an emergency, it can be very important that the hospital knows exactly what's in your system.

A CHECKLIST BEFORE YOU GO INTO THE HOSPITAL

Regardless of whether you are HIV-positive or HIV-negative, hospital stays can be pretty unpleasant and even unhealthy. Too often they offer unappetizing and less-than-nutritious food, lack of exercise and activities, unpleasant sounds, smells, sights, and lighting, and worst of all, complete lack of privacy and personal control. With a little planning, things can be made a lot nicer.

Mark Fotopolis was a friend of mine who was a Broadway actor and was used to making the best of long, national road tours. He applied these techniques to a hospital stay. He had his weekend bag carefully packed the way some would prepare for a short vacation: the perfect combination of toiletries, clothes, Walkman and tapes, address book, and interesting reading.

He moved into his hospital room with colorful (and provocative) posters to brighten up the place, some pink theatrical gel (colored plastic film) to soften one of the fluorescent lighting fixtures, a cheerful blanket to cover the bed, and an oversize teddy bear to keep him company.

He would introduce himself (and the teddy bear) to every staff member who entered his room. He asked politely and said "please" and "thank you" and expected others to do so as well. He called everyone by their first name, not out of disrespect but because he was that sort of friendly person. He wouldn't agree to take one pill or have the simplest of tests unless he understood why and agreed to it.

He spent his time on the phone or writing letters. He visited with other "guests" down the hall and invited old and new friends to join him for lunch and dinner. He asked whoever he could to bring in "real food" from all sorts of places that didn't usually do take-out.

I'm sure he wasn't an easy patient for the

Every now and then go away, have a little relaxation, for when you come back to your work your judgment will be surer; since to remain constantly at work will cause you to lose power of judgment . . . Go some distance away because the work appears smaller and more of it can be taken in at a glance, and a lack of harmony or proportion is more readily seen.

—LEONARDO DA VINCI

hospital staff, but I don't think anyone minded. Here are some ideas to help you make the most of your hospital stay:

- Ask why you are being admitted to the hospital. Could any or all of this be done on an outpatient basis?

- Which hospital will you be going to and why? Ask around at support groups what other people's experiences are with this place regarding people with HIV/AIDS.

- Is this stay for a diagnostic procedure or to treat a medical condition?

- What are the long- and short-term risks associated with this?

- Is it really necessary? If it is a diagnostic procedure, what actions might they take based on the results? Are you prepared and willing to take these actions? If not, then perhaps it's not worth taking the test either. If it's a treatment, what would happen if it were not given? Are there any less "invasive" or risky choices?

- How long do they expect you to stay? What happens if you feel better sooner?

- How often will your doctor visit you? Don't forget to bring your doctor's phone number so you can call directly.

- Does your physician plan to use any "consulting physicians" or other experts? Have you met these folks before?

- How will the finances work? How much is your stay likely to cost? Even if you have insurance, there may be lifetime maximums that you want to be careful about. Will you need any prior authorization from your insurance company or case worker before being admitted?

- How much control will you have? What must you do to review your own chart? Can you request or refuse pain or sleeping medication?

- What are visiting hours? How strict are they about this?

- Sometimes only immediate family is allowed to visit. Do you have a medical power of attorney so that someone other than your relatives can make legal decisions for you if necessary?

- Bring an address book or phone list so if you get bored you have someone you can call.

- Get a telephone credit card. A hospital stay is the perfect time to catch up on old friendships in distant cities, but you can't make long-distance calls without one.

- If your answering machine can be worked by remote control, read the book and figure out how to do it so you can get your messages and change the outgoing message from the hospital. Try it out before you go, and bring the instructions.

- If you expect to be in the hospital for a longer stay, you might change the message on your answering machine so people will call you: "Hi, this is so-and-so. I'm going to be in General Hospital for a few days for tests, and it sure gets BORING over there, so I'd love to hear from you. My number there is 555-0000."

- Don't bring anything valuable with you.

Jewelry must often be removed for tests and surgery. Things have a habit of getting lost or stolen when you're out of the room for a long time.

- You will need a few dollars for TV rental, etc.

- Carefully plan what toiletries you might need. Remember cologne, mouthwash, hair spray, etc. so you can feel clean and attractive even when you're not up for a shower. An electric razor is much easier when you're not feeling well.

- Bring an inexpensive Walkman with a selection of different types of music and meditation tapes. Try books-on-tape so you can catch up on your "reading" even if you don't have the energy to read.

- Bring some colorful and interesting things such as a poster and an attractive blanket to cheer up the room.

WORKING THE SYSTEM

Living with HIV/AIDS is an expensive "hobby" that we all need a little financial help with. At one time or another, this means that you will have to deal with some large bureaucracy, such as an insurance company, hospital, local AIDS services organizations, clinical trial program, or government agency. Here are a few tips to help the process run a little smoother:

- As the old saying goes "you get more flies with honey than you do with vinegar." Don't get angry or yell. It won't get you what you want, and, anyway, it probably wasn't the fault of the person you are talking to that you've been on hold for an hour.

- Be persistent. "The squeaky wheel gets the oil." Be friendly, and be polite, but keep calling.

- If you don't get results, it's really important that you write short, clear letters and demand action. Send copies to other people who might be able to step in and help. When all else fails, don't forget the media and elected officials. Remember that in today's world, never underestimate the power of one person with access to a computer, copier or fax machine.

- Write everything down in your HIV notebook so you can find it next time you call. Get everyone's name and extension or ID number. It will make them more careful and give you some way to follow up. For example "I spoke with Sally Smith at extension 1845 on July 30, and she told me that I didn't need to submit that form . . ."

- Make copies of everything you mail in. That way if it gets lost, or you have to fill out a similar form in the future, you already have everything.

- If you're trying to find out something really important, ask several different people. Often someone will think they know the answer or just make up an answer to get you off the phone.

- Keep businesslike records and files. If you don't have them, buy some home office supplies like file folders and envelopes.

- Make a list of important numbers and keep it in your wallet in case of emergencies. You will need to know your social security number, insurance number, case

*Common sense is
not so common.*
— *VOLTAIRE*

worker's name, doctor's phone number, etc., and it may be difficult to locate them if you unexpectedly find yourself at the hospital or clinic.

- When it's important, confirm everything in writing and get some proof of delivery, such as Federal Express or post office return receipt requested. That way when your payment gets lost, or they claim never to have agreed to something, you can prove them wrong.

- If you have health, disability, or life insurance, make sure the premiums are paid on time. Confirm that they got the payment by phone before the due date, or send it with some proof of delivery, such as Federal Express or post office return receipt requested. The insurance company would love to have a reason to cancel your policy. If you have to, don't pay the rent or utilities, but keep up the insurance. If you simply have no money, try calling the local AIDS services organization; sometimes they have emergency loans for such things.

- If you have any sort of life insurance and are technically diagnosed with a "terminal condition," it may be possible to sell this policy for cash to specialized "viatical settlement companies" who are in the business of purchasing such policies (see "Appendix B" for listings and "Chapter 10" for more information). Instead of your estate or beneficiary receiving money after you die, you may be able to collect as much as 50% to 80% of that amount while you are alive. In effect,

Difficulties are opportunities to better things; they are stepping-stones to greater experience. Perhaps someday you will be thankful for some temporary failure in a particular direction. When one door closes, another always opens; as a natural law it has to, to balance.
—BRIAN ADAMS
How to Succeed

*Health is not a
condition of matter,
but of Mind.*
   —MARY BAKER
        EDDY
   Science and Health

these companies are floating a loan for
some number of months or years, and are
being paid back by the life insurance company, plus a reasonable "interest" at the
time of your death. These companies estimate the discount rate based on how
long they might have to wait to collect
their money. Although this may sound
like a grim option, in fact it can be very
empowering and healthy. HIV/AIDS is expensive and having the cash necessary can
improve both the quality and quantity of
your life. Contact a viatical settlement
company just so you know what sort of
safety net you might have if you need it.

CHAPTER 9

REDUCING STRESS AND GAINING INNER PEACE

> 7 Reduce stress and find daily activities that give you some inner peace and quiet time. Each of us finds serenity in a different way, and only you can know what's right for you. Some people find it through exercise, yoga, or meditation. Others find it by doing something artistic, creative, or by communing with nature. Many enjoy some form of spiritual, religious, or philosophical path.

ABOUT STRESS

Too much stress can kill anyone. It can cause headaches, backaches, stomachaches, ulcers, heart attacks, strokes, and a whole list of very serious conditions and illnesses. Stress also directly reduces the functionality of the immune system.

As they say on late-night TV infomercials, "but wait, there's more." Stress not only causes all sorts of physical problems, it also has a profound mental impact. Daily worries, angers, frustrations, and other sorts of fears build up and rent lots of space in our minds. They prevent the mind from focusing on really important matters; they make you irritable and unpleasant to be around. Stress is just plain bad for you and it doesn't feel good either.

Stress rarely happens all at once. It tends to build up unnoticed slowly over time until the symptoms become so acutely critical that they cannot be avoided.

My philosophy is that not only are you responsible for your life, but doing the best at this moment puts you in the best place for the next moment.

—OPRAH WINFREY

133

It is far easier to deal with the little daily stresses on a regular basis rather than wait until so much has built up to the point that there is a real problem that is difficult to solve.

As unavoidable as stress seems to be in our society, for those of us living with HIV/AIDS, learning to minimize both physical and mental stress can be critical. Even more than in other areas, there is no single answer. Whether one calls it "calmness," "inner peace," "quiet time," or "serenity," different people find it in different ways.

As the song goes "don't worry, be happy." This sounds good, but it can be difficult sometimes to "take it easy," especially when one has to cope with all the stuff that dealing with HIV/AIDS can bring up. Make a conscious effort to put yourself on the "gentle cycle." Each of us has countless important tasks, vital commitments, and pending deadlines, but when you take a moment to think about it, yes, such-and-such may be very important, but is it really worth dying for? Is it really worth literally worrying yourself sick over?

Certainly, it's important to keep your commitments, but at times, we all overcommit ourselves. It doesn't matter how healthy you might be, it's much better to call and say, "I'm really sorry, I really want to, but I overbooked myself, and I just can't" than to make yourself sick trying.

PHYSICAL STRESS MANAGEMENT

Stress certainly has a physical component. You can see stress as physical tension in the muscles of the shoulders, clenched fists and jaw, tight facial muscles, backaches, headaches, digestive problems, ulcers, heart attacks, and strokes. Worst of all for people living with HIV/AIDS, stress greatly reduces the effectiveness of the immune system itself in being able to repair the body and fight disease.

Later in this chapter we will talk about what can

When the lowest vertebrae are plumb erect, the spirit reaches to the top of the head. With the top of the head as if suspended from above. The whole body feels itself light and nimble.

—The Classics of T'ai Chi Ch'uan

cause stress as well as the mental and emotional aspects, but first let's look at the purely physical side of stress.

If you were to hold on to a water glass too lightly, it would fall through your hand, smash on the floor, and make a big mess. Holding on too tightly—with more force than is necessary—has the same effect as holding on with just enough force, except that the muscles are doing more work than necessary. The bad part is it gets to be a habit.

Imagine what it might have been like to live, say, 100,000 years ago. Physically, primitive human beings didn't look all that different back then than we do now. Back then, humans lived pretty much like other animals. They lived and traveled in small packs, hunting and gathering food. They spent most of their time playing, and when the food ran out, they moved on.

Not a bad life. Except at any moment, lions, tigers, and bears (or what have you) could jump out from behind the next bush with a person in mind for their lunchtime treat.

That's where instincts and the central nervous system come in. Even before you see the lion, tiger, or bear (or what have you) you see something in the bushes. Immediately, your body responds: danger!

The body puts everything you have into the life-and-death emergency of getting the large muscle groups ready to fight for your life at almost superhuman strength, or to run away faster than you ever thought you could. All sorts of hormones and chemical signals race throughout your body. You are now ready: Fight or flight.

Unfortunately, your body has limited resources, so to do this it had to stop working on low-priority items like digesting your breakfast, fighting infections, healing old wounds, or even higher-level thinking. As important as these things are, they won't matter if you

I know God will not give me anything I can't handle. I just wish that He didn't trust me so much.
—*MOTHER TERESA*

don't survive the next few minutes. Before you know it, your body decided to run. And run it does. You're safe, and after that emergency workout, your body slowly returns to normal.

In the modern world, lions, tigers, and bears (or what have you) almost never jump out at you. Your body is ready for them anyway. It triggers this same defense system to some degree whenever it perceives or imagines any sort of danger, even abstract mental dangers. The problem is that, say a letter from the IRS or a movie on TV, doesn't give your muscles the opportunity to burn off all this extra energy. After all, when was the last time you actually had to fight or run for your very life?

The result is that your body gets all pumped up with no place to go. The muscles want to work out. That's why when someone gets very angry they will sometimes punch a wall or shake. They have physical energy stored up like a spring ready to explode. Without help, it can be quite difficult for the body to reabsorb all these now-toxic hormones and other chemicals, and tell the various muscle groups and other body parts to relax.

After repeated false alarms, the muscles stay in a state of semireadiness, limiting movement and the free flow of the lymphatic system, and various toxins are stored throughout the body.

The solution is quite simple, although not easy: gently increase muscle flexibility through a combination of massage, acupressure, gentle movement, stretching, regular aerobic workout, and moderate exercise. Cleanse the body by drinking plenty of liquids and eating a healthy diet (see "Chapter 6: Doing Healthy Stuff and Avoiding Unhealthy Stuff").

Some people take the more-physical approach to stress management such as daily stretching, walking, or other aerobic exercise. Other alternatives include the more-formalized physical programs designed for

The great thing in this world is not so much where we stand, but in what direction we are moving.

—OLIVER WENDELL HOLMES

stress management and harmony, such as yoga and T'ai Chi Ch'uan.

Personally, I'm also a fan of massage. Because people with HIV/AIDS are prone to so many unusual skin conditions, I try to take extra good care of my skin: I cleanse out the pores in the steam room, moisturize, and dry everything thoroughly to minimize the possibility of fungal infections such as athlete's foot and jock itch.

PAVLOV'S DOG
The mind associates things that often happen together as being somehow related, even if there is no real connection. To prove this, in 1926, Ivan Pavlov conducted an interesting experiment. He rang a bell just before he fed a dog. The dog came to associate the sound of this bell with getting food, so much so that the dog would drool whenever the bell was rung, even if no food was actually produced.

This phenomenon of Pavlovian Response is very common. I'm sure everyone has had the experience of, for example, getting sick as a kid from eating too much candy corn at Halloween. Now just smelling that candy makes you nauseated. Another example is the smell of a special cologne that reminds you of a certain night. One whiff and your hormones are off and running, even if you're in the elevator at work.

Lee Strasberg, the acting coach who trained Marilyn Monroe, Dustin Hoffman, and Al Pacino, called this phenomenon "Sense Memory" and used it to help actors re-create emotional responses on stage by imagining physical sensations that actually occurred sometime in the actor's past, when he or she experienced a similar emotion or sensation.

We can also use this same phenomenon for stress reduction. Let's say you want to feel healthy, calm, serene, centered, loved, energized, invigorated, vibrant, and safe. What you might do is go to some

Nothing in the world can take the place of persistence. Talent will not; nothing is more common than unsuccessful men with talent. Genius will not; unrewarded genius is almost a proverb. Education will not; the world is full of educated derelicts. Persistence and determination alone are omnipotent.

—CALVIN COOLIDGE

calm place, perhaps a beach or church, and wait around until you feel that way. Then you might do something that acts in the same way as Pavlov's bell. Perhaps you might say a single word (people who meditate call these single words that are repeated over and over again *mantras*) or you might recite the same phrase over and over again, such as "Our father who art in heaven . . ." or any other prayer or ritual. My own personal favorite:

> God, grant me the serenity
> to accept the things I cannot change,
> the courage to change the things I can,
> and the wisdom to know the difference.

Now, the next time you are not feeling at your most safe, serene, calm, or centered, you might repeat that same word or phrase that you have now trained yourself to associate with good things.

On one level, at least, we could say that prayer certainly works. Meditation can be thought of as training your mind to do what you want it to, when you want it to.

Some of you may say, "Wait a minute. Is he trying to say that God does not listen to our prayers, and that it's all some sort of placebo effect?" Prayer means different things to different people. For some, it is a way to talk to God, for others it's a way to listen to an inner voice inside of them. Most people think of a prayer as repeating some written or memorized (words) or activity, but for many prayer is more like a free-form conversation, similar to a meditation.

RELIGION, SPIRITUALITY, AND PERSONAL PHILOSOPHY

It can be very difficult to talk about religion, spirituality, or personal philosophy, because most people feel very strongly about their own position on this subject.

A human being is part of the whole called by us a universe—a part limited in time and space. He experiences himself, his thoughts and his feelings, as something separate from the rest, a kind of optical delusion of his consciousness.

This delusion is a kind of prison for us; it restricts us to our personal decisions and our affections to a few persons nearest to us.

Our task must be to free ourselves from this prison by widening our circle of compassion to embrace all living creatures and the whole of nature in its beauty.

—ALBERT EINSTEIN

Often when someone brings up the subject, they really just want to promote, evangelize, and convert you to his or her own point of view.

Rest assured, I have no wish to change your belief system one bit. I'm not trying to sell you on any one answer. However, dealing with big issues like HIV/AIDS brings up other big issues like mortality, and one's place in the universe. And those questions are addressed by religion, spirituality, and personal philosophy.

There are no right answers, and this book has no agenda to sell you on sticking to or changing your point of view. My only goal is to help you become aware of what you already believe and do not believe in, so that you can make important life choices that are consistent with those beliefs.

Many people dealing with HIV/AIDS and other life-challenging experiences go through a dramatic change in the nature of their religious faith. Some leave a path they have followed for years, and others find comfort in a religion that they haven't thought about since childhood. Many take a long hard look at what they believe and then choose à la carte from traditional sources.

Like most writers, I love to read. One of the most important things about good writing is that it is "internally consistent," meaning that once you accept the things you are asked to believe, for example that vampires are real, or that there are lots of humanlike aliens that we can visit with the Starship *Enterprise*, then everything else makes sense and is believable within that context.

The same is true of your personal belief system. The most important thing is that you are "internally consistent" and that whatever you believe, you behave accordingly. My point is to get you thinking about what you believe. Give yourself permission to disagree with what you were told to believe as a child.

> It is the commonest of mistakes to consider that the limit of our power of perception is also the limit of all there is to perceive.
>
> —C.W. LEADBEATER

I personally get great comfort in feeling that I am an important part of the universe. I know I am not a big piece—no living thing is—and I almost certainly won't have a major impact on the whole, but every piece is significant.

Many people insist that they are nonreligious because they disagree with or do not feel a part of religious traditions that they grew up with.

It certainly is beyond the scope of this book to help you find your own personal enlightenment.

Regardless whether you identify yourself as a Christian, Moslem, Hindu, Buddhist, Taoist, Jew, Atheist, Agnostic, Universalist, or none of these, you do have a personal philosophy or spirituality that may, or that may not, happen to agree with some larger, organized group's.

Spirit is the animating life force within each of us. It is neither sacred nor secular, it just is.

A lot of people have not been well served by religion and in response say that they are not religious or that they don't believe in God. I think it is just that *the form of religion* has changed, and that the very word has gotten a bad rap.

I like to use neutral words instead. For example, I don't like to use the phrase "believe in God" because those words mean so many different things to so many people. Many associate the "G-word" with the religion of their upbringing, which may or may not agree with their current belief system.

MY PERSONAL SPIRITUAL JOURNEY

I would like to take a few pages to explain my own personal spiritual journey for two reasons:

First, although I try to be impartial, my explanations are bound to be colored by my viewpoint; it's important that you understand my bias, so that you can go beyond it to make up your own mind.

Second, whether you agree or disagree with my

philosophy, perhaps the way I explain it will help you, or prod you into a clearer understanding of what *you* believe.

Both my parents grew up in Europe just before World War II. Although both considered themselves Atheists, my mother came from a Lutheran background, and my father from a Jewish background. For them, organized religion was something that separated people into groups of "us" and "them" and caused hostility and intolerance.

Their philosophy at the time was that one of the keys to uniting all the people of the world was to do away with the things that kept them apart. One of these things was organized religion.

As a very small child I was read aloud stories from the Jewish Old Testament, the Christian New Testament, the Moslem Koran, Greek mythology, and fairy tales and folk stories from all over the world. To me, they were all fascinating, but not that different: people walking on water, flying through the air, turning into frogs, or pillars of salt. It wasn't until quite late in school that I learned some people did not view these texts in the same light. In my family, we thought of these people as unscientific, superstitious, ignorant children who were afraid of the dark.

My father was a professor and government advisor, and my mother a political activist. There was always a lot of discussion about morality, ethics, philosophy, social consciousness, the importance of world art, science, history, and culture.

A number of years ago, I joined an atheists' discussion group to clarify how I felt on these issues so that I could plainly say to all those religious nuts, "No, I don't believe in God, I believe such-and-such." I was asked to write a response to what boiled down to the following question: What do you believe happens to "who you are" after you die, and is there anything that is more important than you?

For those who believe, no proof is necessary. For those who don't believe, no proof is possible.
—JOHN AND LYN
ST. CLAIR THOMAS

I took ten pages to answer. My answer is no better or worse than anyone else's, but it is very important to ask the question. I rambled on (and on) that all that I am would live on in the hearts and minds of those who loved me, cared about me, and were affected by me. I wrote that there were lots of things that were more important than I was, everything from all the future generations of people, to the health of the planet, to the cumulative wisdom, creativity, and accomplishments of humanity.

I also talked about faith. I believed that the earth itself is what scientists call a "stable self-renewing system," meaning that it doesn't wear out and that it has built-in forces that correct things when they get out of balance. One might even call it a natural intelligence, in some ways not unlike the human body's immune system.

The universe behaves in certain predictable ways. We describe it as "following laws," but really it's the other way around. Nature behaves whatever way it wants to, and then we humans invent "models" that describe and predict that behavior so that we can better understand and explain it.

I believed that there was a natural balance, rhythm, and flow in the world, and when this was upset, the environment would respond to return the system again to balance. For example, if the population of a certain animal grows too large, lack of food or some other limiting condition brings it back under control.

Today I think the cumulative human experience, understanding, wisdom, and culture is something spiritual and—yes—holy and sacred that needs to be cherished and nurtured.

Equally holy and sacred is our ecosystem: the beautiful "blue marble" called Earth. The natural beauty of a flower or a sunset, the perfect balance of its endless recycling, the infinite variety of life in all its forms, the wonder of human body and mind, and even the miracle of life itself.

Some people like to call these "laws of physics" or "evolution" or "nature's path" or "the immune system," others call them "God's will." I prefer to borrow a term of Eastern philosophy called "Tao," (pronounced more like "Dow" that rhymes with "now") which literally means "the way."

Whether God created these laws or the playing field for them to act in is something I cannot answer. And for this discussion, it is not important.

In the end, I decided that my personal philosophy was a blend of Quaker, Taoist, Native American, Jew, and Universalist.

The Quakers believe that God is in all of us; prayer is getting quiet and listening to that inner voice inside each of us. Since Quakers believe that no one is inherently closer to God, it is a very democratic religion without any permanent ministers or church hierarchy.

The Taoists also believe that there is no external God, but there is a natural balance or path. Again, prayer is viewed as listening for "The Way."

The Native American's spirituality is based on the idea that the Mother Earth herself is a living being, and that humans and all other animals are her children.

The Universalist sees all religious and spiritual options as being different paths up the same mountain. The higher up one goes, the more they converge into a single path, finally leading to the same destination.

The Jews believe that Truth is found through the academic and philosophical teaching, study, and discussion of the cumulative works of man and God.

I know that I am more than just my body. My personality, creativity, and love are more than merely intellectual thoughts: I do not know if this emotional-creative energy (which others have called the

I simply haven't the nerve to imagine a being, a force, a cause which keeps the planets revolving in their orbits, and then suddenly stops in order to give me a bicycle with three speeds.
—QUENTIN CRISP

spirit) exists apart from the body, but this is not important. My spirit does exist now. I am not my body, I am my spirit. I know that this spirit can be nurtured through practicing love and creativity, as well as other spiritual exercises such as meditation and group processes.

For me group processes are particularly important because they show me that my spirit can be joined with other people's spirits and blossom. A loving group of people creates more love. Smiles are infectious. A group of artists or intellectuals is more creative collectively than individually.

For me, today, God is that little voice within myself and everyone else that is loving, creative, and good. When I was a little child my mother told me that "God" was merely an abbreviation for "good."

Learning to listen to that still quiet inner voice also means trusting that it is worth listening to. The louder voices—those of the ego—have all the rational arguments. It takes faith to listen to the quiet voices and follow them when rational arguments disagree.

I do not believe in any God that rewards or punishes us, but I do believe that there are consequences for our actions, and that we are free to take whatever actions we want. If we do not follow our Tao, it's like swimming upstream. We may get where we want, but not without a lot of unnecessary effort.

This has allowed me to remember that there is something greater than myself. We live in a world where it is particularly easy to become totally selfish. "What's in it for me and mine?" has become the catchphrase of the era.

I do not pretend to be a Mother Teresa or Einstein, but today I do remember to quote history's most famous man in his Sermon on the Mount: "Do unto others as you would have them do unto you."

I also know that our home is a small planet: we

can no longer afford to foul our own nests. Being socially responsible begins with me.

This is my personal view—and again, this is what I believe, not what is "true" or what you should believe.

Many people who might insist that they do not have any religious or spiritual path are actively involved, or even driven to doing something that they feel is very important.

The purpose is to connect with your life force, and certainly expressing yourself, in any creative way, does just that. Perhaps this connection may have nothing to do with your concept of God or of the universe, but it nonetheless is based on your spirit.

Now that we have grounded ourselves, and plugged into whatever belief system is appropriate for us, let's tackle the last big hurdle, facing life and death . . .

If one is master of one thing and understands one thing well, one has at the same time, insight into and understanding of many things.
—VINCENT
VAN GOGH

CHAPTER 10

SIMPLIFYING AND REEVALUATING LIFE AND DEATH

> **8** Life is a process of growth and change. Along the way, each of us has developed our own unique "survival kit" to cope with whatever stuff we needed to. We carry with us the scars and baggage from this process. It's important not only to pick up new experiences, ideas, possessions, friends, and new ways of looking at things, but also to edit out the old ones that no longer work for us.
>
> This "spring cleaning" process of simplifying life and reevaluating goals, priorities, and beliefs is seldom easy—particularly when the big issues are family, finances, career, material possessions, life's purpose, and even our own mortality—but it can be incredibly rewarding and liberating.

LIFE IS A PROCESS OF GROWTH AND CHANGE

If you're into guilt you're playing God. The universe is created so it's O.K. to make a mistake. If you feel guilty about what you have done, you're saying it's not O.K. to make mistakes.

—SUSAN HAYWARD

The person we have become is largely determined by how we have interacted with our environment, what we have experienced, and the thoughts and emotions of a lifetime. Because of the physical way that the body and the mind work, we cannot think or do anything without being changed by that thought or action. The mind is literally made up of these learned mental associations.

Things we practice—even bad habits—usually become easier, more comfortable, and more pleasurable the more we do them. Actions that once caused

146

unpleasant results—or that we believe to cause un-pleasant reactions—tend to bring up unpleasant memories and sensations to discourage us from doing them again.

Unfortunately, the mind sometimes learns the wrong lesson. It doesn't always make the best mental associations. If you watch a sexy girl or guy on TV next to a can of soda often enough, most people will start to associate that soda with sex. On one level, your mind knows that the two have nothing to do with one another, but on another level, it thinks they do, and that's why advertising is a lucrative and pervasive part of our culture.

The whole of science is nothing more than a refinement of everyday thinking.
—ALBERT EINSTEIN

In order to grow, we must first admit the need to change, admit that perhaps some other alternative might be better. We risk being wrong. It is very important to be wrong. If you're never wrong, then you aren't trying new things. When one is living with HIV/AIDS, this attitude is trouble.

Having made less than the best choices in the past is a positive growth experience and not something to be ashamed of. Buckminster Fuller put it this way:

Do not fear mistakes. There are none.
—MILES DAVIS

Humans have learned only through mistakes. The billions of humans in history have had to make quadrillions of mistakes to have arrived at the state where we now have 150,000 common words to identify the many unique and only metaphysically comprehensible nuances of experience.

Chagrin and mortification caused by their progressively self-discovered quadrillions of errors would long ago have given humanity such an inferiority complex that it would have become too discouraged to continue with the life experience.

To avoid such a proclivity humans were designedly given pride, vanity, and inventive memory, which, all together, can and usually do incline us to self-deception.

So effective has been the non-thinking, group deceit of humanity that it now says, "Nobody should make mistakes," and punishes people for making mistakes. The courage to adhere to the truth as we learn it involves, then, the courage to face ourselves, with the clear admission of all the mistakes we have made— mistakes are sins only when not admitted.

REEVALUATING YOUR LIFE-STYLE

One of the most important factors in enjoying one's life is to find a life-style that feels right and that works for you. Some people think of "life-style" as a code word meaning only sexual preference, or living arrangement, or career choice, but it's all these things, and hundreds more. What do you eat and drink? Do you live alone or with a group or with someone special? Do you live in the city or the country? Do you work for one person or company or many . . . or none? How do you spend your time and money? What is your life's purpose?

When I look at my life's purpose, it boils down to enjoying my life, helping others to enjoy theirs, and doing my best to clean up my own mess and leave the world a little better because I passed through. For me, that's what life's all about: each generation building on the accomplishments of the one before.

When I was in high school, I read Henry David Thoreau's *Walden* and it had a profound impact on my life. Thoreau's basic tenet was that we could be much happier in our lives if we lived deliberately. We should look at how much pleasure we got out of material things and what it cost us in terms of time, effort, and unpleasantness to purchase those things.

The book did not offer any answers, it merely raised the question of how much pleasure per dollar you gain from "things" and how much pain per dollar it costs you to earn enough to pay for it.

Would you rather work six days a week and live

Work is love made visible.
—KAHLIL GIBRAN
The Prophet

The cost of a thing is the amount of what I call life which is required to be exchanged for it, immediately or in the long run.
—HENRY DAVID THOREAU

Money doesn't always bring happiness. People with ten million dollars are no happier than people with nine million dollars.
—HOBART BROWN

in a beautiful house or work only two days a week and live in a simple rented room? Perhaps you would trade a job you hate for a job you love where you only make half as much.

REEVALUATING YOUR MATERIAL POSSESSIONS

I have helped clean out half a dozen friends' homes after they have died, and the experience has taught me a lot. Things just aren't that important. Even the most valuable things get broken, lost, stolen, or sold. Most of a person's treasures that were once so meaningful to them just become so much ugly, useless trash. In the end, only the intangibles really count.

The wise man does not lay up treasure; his riches are within. The more he gives to others, the more he has of his own.
—LAO-TZU

I'm one of those people who fill up a whole page in my friends' address books. I don't think I've ever stayed in one place for more than about 18 months. I don't think I've ever met anyone who likes to move, but it certainly does have its advantages.

It's a great opportunity to go through all your stuff and figure out what's worth packing up and making space for, what to give away, and what stuff has outlived its usefulness. I like to live in big cities and on the beach, both places where every inch of space is expensive, so I can't afford not to sort things out. Moving can also be a time to make a fresh start and change some of the less-tangible things that you have not been happy with in your life. Perhaps this is why so many people hate moving so much, because it drags out all the junk from their lives that they have worked so hard to hide away.

If something hasn't been useful or given me joy within the last year, then it probably isn't important for who I am today. Like all rules, there are exceptions. The IRS wants financial records back seven years and I do have some boxes of memorabilia, keepsakes, and old photographs that I only occasionally go through.

There must be more to life than having everything!
—MAURICE SENDAK

Our possessions can give us great joy, or they

can be a great burden. Sometimes they help define our place in the universe, linking us with history and the future. The key is to find the balance between the two.

REEVALUATING YOUR SECRETS

The trouble with the
rat race is that even
if you win, you're
still a rat.
—LILY TOMLIN

Living with secrets doesn't feel very good. It is full of fear and lies, and can choke the very life force out of you. In the early years of HIV/AIDS there was a very politically incorrect joke that went "What's the worst thing about having AIDS? It's telling your parents that you're Haitian." The truth is that most of the time, living with HIV/AIDS does not show, and the average person on the street will assume that you are HIV-negative.

This causes all sorts of problems. To whom should you disclose that you are living with HIV/AIDS? Your family, your employer, your friends, your neighbors, your sexual partners? How about your insurance company and other institutions that you deal with? Who do you tell, and when and how do you tell them?

It's a sad fact that even after over a dozen years of public education, being openly HIV-positive has such a strong stigma attached to it that for some it could destroy family and career if it were disclosed improperly. Probably the best advice for now is not to tell anyone outside your closest loved ones for a while, until you've thought things through and planned things out a bit. Once you let the news out, you have no control of where it goes, and you have to be prepared for the consequences.

Most people who become HIV infected today do so through sexual activity or recreational injection drug use, neither of which are subjects that most of us feel comfortable talking about openly. Sometimes disclosing one's HIV status brings up discussions of marital infidelity, a history of recreational injection drug use, or homosexuality.

It can also bring up a whole host of irrational fears: the general population still doesn't have a clear understanding that HIV can only be transmitted through extremely intimate circumstances. Most people are also afraid of being around someone who may be dealing with mortality because it brings up their own.

In almost ten years of attending HIV/AIDS support groups, the question of hiding and disclosing one's HIV status is without a doubt the single most talked- and worried-about issue. Each person must find what's right for him or her in each situation, and sometimes it takes months of talking and planning before someone becomes ready to let go and share the news.

The amazing part is that in almost all the cases, after the initial shock, the results were almost always unbelievably supportive, with friends, families, and employers rising to the occasion. Even the people who you would have thought the last people on earth to be able to handle it, responded with love and support beyond wild expectations. Of course, there have been a handful of rejections in all that time, but usually, only temporary ones.

I'd like to share with you some of the more remarkable successes.

JIM'S STORY

Jim came from a born-again Christian family from Texas and worked in New York for one of the largest computer software firms. Having AIDS was his deepest secret. He scheduled lunchtime doctor's appointments, took vacation days to hide hospital visits, and did whatever he had to so that no one at the office would guess. All this was quite a strain on him.

When he finally was forced to tell his employer, he was sure that it would be the end of his career. Nothing could have been farther from the truth.

That software company couldn't have been more

My religion is very simple—my religion is kindness.
—THE DALAI LAMA

White people think that you are your work...Black people think that my work is just what I have to do to get what I want.
—MARY ANNE MADISON

supportive. They gave him a flexible schedule and an assistant to take over some of his responsibilities so he could keep working on the "fun stuff." Subsequently, Jim helped roll out two new products. The software company got a pretty good deal; the benefit of Jim's expertise as well as a thoroughly trained replacement.

When Jim chose to move back to Texas to be with his family for those last few months, the company relocated him to the Texas office—complete with a new office and new business cards. I don't know how much work he did down there before he died, but it was certainly a classy way to reward five years of loyal service.

JOHN'S STORY

It took me four years to paint like Raphael, but a lifetime to paint like a child.
—*PABLO PICASSO*

John Jones is a high school art teacher at the Friends Seminary, a Quaker-founded school in New York. The following letter tells his story better than I could:

November 15, 1992

Dear Parents and Students,

In 1986 I finished my first year of teaching at Friends Seminary totally exhausted. Most of us did, as that was our big bicentennial, and we were all involved in many wonderful activities. However I felt more exhausted than I wanted to be. Doctors visits followed, and on June 20, 1986 I was told that I was HIV-positive. Six weeks later, as a result of the virus, I was in hospital undergoing surgery to remove my spleen. In August I returned to teaching scared, weak, and very nervous . . . and also the keeper of an enormous "secret." I certainly did not feel comfortable telling people what was going on. I did not lie, but instead I did not tell the whole truth.

An incredible journey of tremendous emotional and spiritual growth began to accelerate at this time. Life took on a whole new meaning. My values and priorities changed. It was, and continues to be, a very exciting journey.

Slowly I began to share my "secret" with family and friends. With each sharing, a great weight lifted from my shoulders and a tremendous amount of love and support flowed into my life.

Three years ago, on the last day of the school year, I nervously told my teaching colleagues. The outpouring of love, encouragement, and inspiration from them was totally overwhelming and again a weight from my shoulders lifted.

It has become obvious to me that keeping silent is not my path. Perhaps I have been to too many memorial services and scratched too many names from my address book to remain quiet.

Today I am heavily involved working in the AIDS community, which is not a separate community, but a community that belongs to all of us. I find this work both rewarding and heartbreaking.

So the time seemed finally appropriate to let the last group of people, the parents and students of Friends Seminary in on my "secret." Now my "secret" is no more, and for me much fear, anxiety, and projection is washed away.

Today I am not only committed to my art teaching, but also to educating our children about the world of AIDS we all live in. For the first time I now feel I can accomplish this with

A Hasid asked his Rebbe: "How can I best serve God?" expecting to hear a profound and esoteric answer. The Rebbe replied: "One can best serve God with whatever one is doing at the moment."
—*Hasidic Teaching*

my heart open and coming from a totally honest position.

Thank you very much to Rich, the ad-
ministrative staff, the faculty, and staff. I hope
you realize how truly amazing your support has
been.

I believe that the times ahead will be exciting and rewarding for all of us.

Thank you.

Much love,
John Jones

The most wonderful part of this story is the
overflowing scrapbook of wonderful, supportive, loving
letters that John received from the parents, telling him
how fortunate they are that he is teaching their children. Not one person reacted negatively, or asked to
have their child moved, which says quite a lot about
the quality of people at the Friends Seminary.

A PRACTICAL GUIDE TO DEATH AND DYING

As a society, one of our biggest fears and taboo subjects is death. Most of us find it very difficult to talk
plainly when it comes to mortality. We avoid the topic
because it's bad manners, bad luck, or both. Even the
most rational and scientific of us are almost superstitious when we talk about death.

We use pleasant-sounding euphemisms such as
"he is no longer with us" as if someone had moved
to a far-off city. We say polite phrases like "*if you
were to die*" as if it might be possible that *you might
not die.* As a society, we don't like to think about it.
We don't want to talk about it. And we certainly do
not want to make plans. All this just reenforces our

*I am indeed rich,
since my income is
superior to my
expense, and my
expense is equal to
my wishes.*

*—EDWARD
GIBBON*

*Man fears death as
children fear to go
in the dark; and as
that natural fear in
children is increased
with tales, so is the
other.*

*—SIR FRANCIS
BACON*

fear of death. After all, *we are all going to die*, the only question is when.

For those of us living with a life-challenging condition such as HIV/AIDS, this taboo can be particularly strong. Often we find the very idea of planning for our own eventual death, or for the death of someone we care about, as somehow giving up—as accepting defeat of HIV/AIDS as a fatal disease. Nothing could be farther from the truth. Hiding from those fears only makes them worse, confronting them head-on conquers them.

FUNERALS AND MEMORIALS ARE FOR THE LIVING

Coping with the loss of someone you care about is one of the most difficult things that one ever has to go through. It is the subject of many books all by itself. In fact, there are a number of wonderful books on exactly this subject in "Appendix A: Suggested Reading" under the twin sections *The Practical Side of Death, Dying, and Grief* and *The Emotional Side of Death, Dying, and Grieving.*

Death is nothing to us, since when we are, death has not come, and when death has come, we are not.

—EPICURUS

Funerals and memorials are not for the dead, they are for the living. They serve a very real, practical purpose, and can be a vitally important part of the grieving process. They bring together people who are all experiencing the varying degrees of the same heartbreak. They provide an opportunity for closure, and for people to give support to one another, to validate their feelings, to reenforce their memories, and to find comfort as a part of the larger, ongoing history of mankind.

It's difficult for most of us to view death as a natural and wonderful part of life, because the rhythm of life and death takes so very long, and all of us are alive for such a very short time—compared to the history of humanity. For me, this is the issue that each of us seeks an answer to with our own personal spiritual, religious, or philosophical belief system: understanding the rhythm of life and death and our personal relationship to the universe.

For me, I think nature—or God, or what have you—knows what it's doing. The rhythm of life and death is not unlike the rhythm of changing seasons. The rebirth of spring is followed by the carefree days of summer, then the autumn harvest, and then the apparent death of winter, only to be followed by the rebirth of spring in an endless cycle.

In primitive times, winter was a very scary time. The whole earth dried up and died. This is why all cultures and all religions celebrate the changing seasons, and almost universally they all celebrate a festival of lights in the darkest days of winter, reminding everyone of the rhythm of the seasons. It is for this same purpose that these religions and cultures all celebrate birth, adulthood, marriage, and death. They help us to see the continuity of life itself.

MEMORABLE MEMORIALS

Over the years I have attended dozens of funerals and memorials. Some of them have been wonderful, and others, well frankly, they were pretty dreadful. The purpose of funerals and memorials is to help and comfort those who will attend them, and since different people have different needs, each takes on a different character.

One of the nicest memorials—if you can call a memorial nice—was for my friend Christopher, who was a schoolteacher. He was cremated without any sort of funeral, and shortly after his death, I got this wonderful, formal invitation to a dinner party at his home.

When I got there, it was filled with all sort of folks I hadn't seen in years. His favorite music was on the stereo, home movies were playing on the TV, and on every surface and by every seating area, there were photo albums of all the times we had all shared with Christopher. We told stories, and laughed—and cried, and laughed some more.

We were given a gift of a small booklet containing a wonderful photo of him and some poems he had picked out before he died. We were handed pieces of paper and asked to write a short note to our departed friend. We tied these notes onto balloons, and all walked down to the shore holding on to the strings like little children at an amusement park.

When we got to the water's edge, some people sang or played recorded music, and others told a few last stories of what he had been like as a teacher, a lover, a dance buddy, and theater nut.

As the sun set, we let go of our balloons (that was before we knew of the bad effects they can have on marine life) and watched them disappear into the cloudless sky. That was such a wonderful last memory of my friend.

Personally I tend to like this sort of nontraditional, participatory memorial service rather than a religious funeral, but not long ago I attended John's funeral, which reminded me how comforting cultural traditions can be for those who grew up with them.

John came from a conservative, Italian Catholic neighborhood, and his family naturally arranged a traditional funeral: open casket wake, Catholic mass, and in-ground cemetery burial. Propped up in the casket, he certainly looked at peace, and almost happy. This was a much nicer way to remember him than he had looked just a few days before. For those who couldn't believe that he was dead, this certainly was convincing.

Friends and family returned to the very church that many of them had attended as children, had been married in, and had their own children baptized in. They all knew when to stand up, when to sit down, when to kneel, and what words to repeat after the priest. After the final rites at the cemetery, most peo-

We do not know whether it is good to live or to die. Therefore, we should not take delight in living nor should we tremble at the thought of death. We should be equal minded towards both. This is the ideal.

—MAHATMA GANDHI

ple went to visit a few other graves. All this gave such a feeling of continuity, of death as a normal part of life.

A MOTHER'S TRIBUTE
Memorials are not just alternative funeral ceremonies. My dear friend Mark Fotopolis was a Broadway dancer. He always sent out the most wonderful Christmas letters so all his friends could catch up on his travels and adventures.

It seems to me most strange that men should fear; Seeing that death, a necessary end, Will come when it will come.

—WILLIAM SHAKESPEARE

Shortly after he died, I got a Christmas letter from his mother, who lovingly told of all the happiness and joy they had shared in that last year together. She enclosed a photo of her son that I cherish, taken shortly before his death. Naturally, he wasn't physically what he once had been, but it showed someone who had kept his joy and love of life, even when facing death. Let me share this letter with you.

Christmas, 1991

Dear Friends,

Knowing that so many of you look forward to Mark's Christmas letter, I thought I would send it for him this year.

For those of you who have not yet heard, Mark died on November 29th after 6 years and 7 months of living courageously with aids (remember he said that to write aids in capital letters placed greater importance on it than it deserved. "Caps" were to be used for words like LOVE and JOY). Mark spent a lot of 1991 in the hospital or recuperating between hospital visits. He used to joke that he would get to know every hospital in San Francisco. Well, they got to know him in four of them and he captured the hearts of the staff and brightened the days for many fellow patients. Mark's sister Paula spent several months with him in California. The two of them were very close and she was definitely the best medicine in the world for him! His father, stepmother, and I were at his side as often as possible as were so many of his friends. His sister Kate and brother Peter kept in touch at all times showing their love through phone calls and tapes.

In late August, the flat Mark and Tim shared was sold and Mark was faced with the decision of where to relocate. By September, he had settled in with his father in Fernandina Beach, Florida where he and his dog Lucky were able to enjoy sunny days walking along the shores of the Atlantic. Marcia, his stepmother, threw him a gala 35th birthday party September 25th, reminiscent of his first Broadway show, "A Chorus Line," complete with silver and gold balloons and high hats. She invited me to be his "surprise present" and he was truly surprised as I had called him from Downers Grove that morning to wish him a Happy Birthday. It was a loving experience for both of us. Later, we talked about death and dying, holding each other and crying. I told Mark he would have to tell me when he had enough of getting stuck with needles, chemotherapy and all its side effects, and fighting the disease. He would have to tell me it was time to "let go," just as he had done for his good friend Eddie Stone before Eddie died.

In October, Kate spent a few days with him. They had a special spiritual bonding. I spent a week with Mark when Kate left while his Dad and Marcia were in Boston. We enjoyed our walks on the beach and quiet times together. It was fun to be able to cook his fa-

I do want to get rich, but never want to do what there is to do to get rich.
—GERTRUDE STEIN

vorite foods. His appetite never ceased to amaze me! He was feeling so well that he planned a trip to New York where he visited with many of his friends and got to see three Broadway shows. He tired easily, but said he had a wonderful time.

On November 27th, Mark went into the hospital for the last time. I was in Connecticut when his father and Marcia called me and I took the first flight to Jacksonville Thanksgiving morning. Mark always said, "Thanks for coming, Mom" each time I flew to be at his side, and they were his first words when we hugged each other. Despite his labored breathing and other problems, he was able to enjoy a wonderful turkey dinner that Marcia had prepared for him. (I told you he had a great appetite!)

Friday evening, after hours of kidney dialysis, Mark and I were alone and he said to me, "Mom, is it time to let go?" It was time and I told him, "Yes, if you think so." We shared some precious moments and a little later, after a phone call, I was able to tell him that a dear friend of his was expecting twins in July. He smiled that wonderful smile and said, "Oh, that's great!" His father and Marcia joined us again and his Dad told him to close his eyes and take a nap, and the three of us left his room. Mark chose to leave us in the brief time we were gone.

My thanks to Tim, Robert, and his many other friends for the love, care, and support they gave him. With their help Mark was a shining example of courage to others living with aids. His light will always shine in our hearts! I know Mark would want to wish each of you

There is no cure for birth and death save to enjoy the interval.
—GEORGE SANTAYANA

a joyous holiday season as I, and his family, do also.

With love,
Anne Beckmann

EMPTY CHAIRS AT EMPTY TABLES

One of the disadvantages of living so long in a world with HIV/AIDS is losing so many friends, family, lovers, and other heroes along the way. According to a June 1994 *Newsweek* poll, 84% of Americans personally know at least one person who has died from AIDS, and 19%—almost 1 out of every 5 Americans—know more than 20 people who have died from AIDS.

Death is not the greatest loss in life. The greatest loss is what dies inside us while we live.
—NORMAN COUSINS

This never ending, cumulative grief builds up and can be toxic if you don't find a way to process it. For me, the key has been to turn this grief into the motivational force to try to make things a little better. This has been one of the key motivating factors in writing this book and the rest of my work with the HIV/AIDS community.

Often, it can be the grief for losing all those faces that make up the background of our lives: the familiar hug at a support group, a smile from a favorite waiter, the warm hello from a local shopkeeper. Too often I never did know their names. Fran Peavey, a wonderful woman living with HIV wrote in her book, *A Shallow Pool of Time*:

> Fall 1987—It is the strangest thing, but I am beginning to miss people. Not anyone I knew personally, for the most part, but people who were always part of the neighborhood landscape. The two men in shorts at church are gone now. I don't know where they are. Joe Robertson isn't around anymore. Some of the regulars on the street have just disappeared. The change is almost imperceptible—it's as if the ghosts of these people

are hovering around, reminding me that they're gone. Are they all dead? I don't know and can't figure out who or how to ask. I tried calling Joe once but got an answering machine, and he didn't return my call. So he must still be alive. But I have a very distinct feeling that people are just dropping out of existence.

Not knowing who's alive and dead or if anyone else is left who remembers an absent friend is difficult. That's one of reasons for the Vietnam War Memorial. It's also one of the wonderful things about The NAMES Project.

THE NAMES PROJECT

Another nontraditional memorial is The Names Project, a gigantic quilt made up of separate three-foot-by-six-foot sections, each lovingly made for someone who has died from HIV/AIDS by someone who loves and misses them. As of August 1994, there were over 27,000 panels, weighing a total of 37 tons, and when displayed in full, it covers 16 football fields. Even at this mind-boggling size, The Quilt only represented about 12% of the quarter million AIDS death in the United States so far.

In addition to The Quilt itself, The Names Project has a tradition of people reading the names—beginning with "I remember . . ."—of those who have died from HIV/AIDS. This is a very powerful and empowering tradition. When I first heard this reading of The Names, it was in Washington, DC, and the number of Americans killed by AIDS had just exceeded the number of Americans killed in the Vietnam War. Since then, there are now five times that many.

On our way back to our hotel, we walked past the Vietnam War Memorial Wall, and we were all struck by the chilling similarities and the differences of these twin memorials. Michael Callen, inspirational activist, singer, and AIDS survivor of a dozen plus years who died in 1993 used to sing: "We are living in war time/It will not go away/More die every day/This is war . . ."

I'd like to share with you my own list, because without them, I wouldn't be here today, and certainly this book could not exist. Whenever I read it, I like to think of all of those wonderful faces of people whose names I never knew, and all the countless others who I've been cheated out of ever having in my life.

If I have seen further, it is by standing upon the shoulder of Giants.
—*SIR ISAAC* NEWTON

I REMEMBER . . .

Alan Kanghi; Aldyn McKean; Alison Gertz; Alvin Ailey; Anthony Luisi, Jr.; Anthony Perkins; Arthur Ashe; Artie Felson; Barry T. Bragg; Bill Crosby; Bill Giammarese; Bob Harrington; Bob Lewis Schwartzman; Bobby Mondrus; Bruce Mailman; Chaka Savalis; Charles Ludlum; Charles Terrel; Christopher Noel Cross; Christopher Wells; Clovis Ruffin; Curt Davis; Dale Bailey; Dan Hartman; David Burns; David Haney; David Kirchenbaum; David Lee; David Scott Sayles; Derek Jarman; Erinne Hartfield; Ethyl Eichelberger; Fransico "Paco'" Martinez-Cancel; Freddie "Mercury" Bulsara; Gary LeDonne; George-Paul Rosell; Giovanni Richetti; Greg Koulis; Greg Porto; Halston; Haui Montogue; Henry Winslow; Jacques Morali; James Kirkwood; James Revson; Jason Cohen; Jeffrey Schmalz; Jerry Doff; Jerry Gabrielle; Jim Boduszek; Jim Simonette; Joe Nunez; Joey Welsh; John Blanda; John Boswell; Jürgen Honeyball; Keith Haring; Kenn Duncan; Kevin Grubb; Kieran Liscoe; Lawrence Biris; Leonce Chabernaud; Lew Feldman; Liberace; Louis Martinez; Lynne Carter; Malcomb West; Mark Fotopolis; Martin Patrick Gallagher, Jr.; Marty Lipton; Michael "Eve" Fletcher; Michael Barry; Michael Bennett; Michael Biamby; Michael Callen; Michael Hansen; Michael Hirsch; Michael Pappas; Michael Rock; Paul M. Geib; Pedro Zamora; Perry Ellis; Peter Allen; Randy Shilts; Richard Long; Richard Parissidi; Robert Joffrey; Robert La Tourneaux; Robert Mapplethorpe; Rock Hudson; Ron Berst; Ross Johnson; Ru-

dolph Nureyev; Ryan White; Sarah Anne Powers;
Sharon Redd; Shaun Buchanan; Shighiko Nishiguchi
(Nishi); Stanley Berke; Stanley Roman; Stark Hassel-
tine; Steve Rubel; Steve Seifert; Steven Cohn; Stewart
McKinney; Sylvester; Tim Ryan; TJ Myers; Tom
Arminio; Tom Waddell; Tripper Dell; Vinnie Falco;
Vito Russo; Wayland Flowers and Madam; Wil Garcia;
Willi Smith; William Avington; and Zahid Mahmood.

THINGS TO AVOID

Personally, I have witnessed countless horror stories,
all of which could have been avoided with so very little
effort. I want to share some of these with you, so that
you can see the importance to taking the simple actions that we will discuss in this section.

*Death and taxes
and childbirth!
There's never any
convenient time for
any of them.*
—SCARLETT
O'HARA

Anthony's whole life was in Manhattan, but his
funeral wasn't. It was in a faraway hometown, the very
place that he had been so eager to escape from so
many years before. His family didn't think to invite
any of his friends, although a few found out anyway.
Mainly the church was attended by a few distant relatives who probably hadn't sent a Christmas card in
years—if ever.

His death was naturally attributed to "cancer,"
anything other than HIV/AIDS. Well-meaning family
friends wrote out checks to the American Cancer Society. All the things and people that were important
to my friend, all his accomplishments, were hidden
and covered up, and replaced with a preprinted service
suitable for anyone. Of course the gossip I overheard
at the wake was that everyone knew it was AIDS—but
because it was never spoken, the family felt so very
alone in bearing this tragedy.

Back in 1985 I called Bill to ask him if he were
going out dancing at The Saint that night. A strange
voice answered and told me that he had died almost
a month before. I have been cheated out of so many

opportunities to say good-bye and to grieve over the loss of so many friends, because no one knew whom to contact, or how.

These days, I almost assume anyone I haven't heard from in a while must have died, or at least gotten sick and disappeared back to their old hometown, which sometimes is worse . . .

I have said good-bye to Barry, a former business partner, who had wasted away to 90 pounds, and was at peace about his imminent death, only to learn that a year later he was still alive. Against all his wishes, his family moved him to a Midwestern hospital and insisted that any and all efforts be used to "save" him.

Another business partner of mine, Steven, was so afraid that his reputation (and his business) would be ruined if gossip of his condition leaked out, that he insisted to everyone—including his very best friends—that he was HIV-negative.

He attributed his repeated hospitalizations for obvious HIV/AIDS complications to some undiagnosable, mystery disease, that just happened to be treated by prominent HIV/AIDS specialists. Naturally, all this fooled no one, but out of politeness, we all pretended that it did. Eventually, he could no longer continue with this cover-up, so he chose to disappear to Florida, cutting off all contact with his friends and the outside world.

Karen was prohibited from visiting her lover in the hospital, and then locked out of the home they had built together for ten years by well-meaning Southern parents who didn't understand why this "roommate" was so upset about being told she had to move out.

When Bob died over eight years ago, he left things in such disarray, that today the estate still has not been sorted out, his friends and family have all been driven apart over petty arguments, and any money that might have gone to people he cared about,

Lack of money is the root of all evil.
—GEORGE BERNARD SHAW

instead went to the accountants and lawyers. When I think of him, quite frankly, most of the time I think of sorting out all that junk and the endless paperwork and legal battles.

PLANNING AHEAD

Planning ahead and having the right legal paperwork completed can make the whole process so much easier. For example, writing even the simplest of wills, even if you don't have anything worth leaving to anybody, will save those left behind all sorts of bureaucratic night-mares. Without the right legal paperwork, many options such as hospital visits, refusal of extraordinary medical measures, and even cremation can be almost impossible.

Unfortunately, most people die without ever hav-ing made a will, a living will, or even expressing their wishes for their final arrangements. Often funerals and memorials don't meet the needs of those who would benefit from attending them. This is too bad, and sometimes it can be catastrophic.

Not planning ahead needlessly makes things so very much more difficult for those left behind. One of my really important goals in life is to leave things in such a way as to make it simple and as easy as possible for my friends and family to go on after I'm gone.

Money will come to you when you are doing the right thing.
—MICHAEL PHILIPS

It's so simple that most people don't even need a lawyer for any of this. The least expensive option is purchasing blank forms from any stationery store for a couple of bucks and filling them out carefully, and having them signed and witnessed properly. Most local AIDS services organizations can also help prepare these documents. For information about living wills and eu-thanasia, contact a national advocacy organization such as Choice in Dying or The Hemlock Society (see "Appendix B: National and Regional Resources").

Naturally, these documents won't do any good if no one knows that they exist. The originals should be stored in a safe place at home. Although not legally required, it's best if the people who are affected by these documents receive a copy, particularly your doctor, immediate family, and lawyer. This avoids all sorts of problems and conflicts that might otherwise crop up later on.

If you have a computer, the simplest option by far is to use WillMaker 5, computer software from Nolo Press for Macintosh, Windows, and DOS. WillMaker asks you a series of simple questions and prepares a legal will, living will (health-care directive), and documents your wishes for your funeral or other final arrangements.

To be clever enough to get a great deal of money, one must be stupid enough to want it.
—GEORGE BERNARD SHAW

LAST WILL AND TESTAMENT

If you were to die without having a legal will, state laws determine—depending on your legal state of residence at the time of your death, *as listed on the death certificate*—who would inherit whatever money, assets, and other possessions you may have at the time of your death *that are left over* after all your debts and taxes are paid.

Usually these laws follow a pretty self-explanatory chain: *all of* your residual assets would go to your legal husband or wife (but not domestic partner), even if you were legally separated but not divorced. If you did not have a living husband or wife, then your assets would go to your children, parents, or siblings (brothers and sisters), or other relatives in that order.

Some assets—such as the proceeds from a life insurance and jointly owned bank accounts and property—go directly to the beneficiary or co-owner, and are therefore not part of the estate and are not included in a will.

Having an up-to-date will is very important, even if you do not have any significant assets, or if your wishes are the same as what the law would do without a will. A will appoints a *personal representative*, also called an executor (if it's a male) or executrix (if it's a female). This *personal representative* is able to make all sorts of decisions and to take actions. For example, some types of funeral arrangements can be difficult or even impossible without such specific authority. Estates of people with wills are settled much faster and with much less paperwork than those without them.

A will also allows you to divide whatever money, assets, and other possessions you may have at the time of your death and give them to the people or organizations of your choosing. A will can also serve several other very important functions. A will can "forgive" debts, meaning that someone who owes you money won't have to pay it back. It also expresses how outstanding debts, funeral expenses, and taxes should be paid.

Although a legal will is best, even an informal note will help others know what you wanted. If you want to give something to someone after you're gone, write it down.

Often, because of large debts, for example large medical expenses, there may be more debts than there are assets. If this is the case, then there are no assets *left over* after all your debts and taxes are paid, and therefore there is nothing that can be inherited, regardless of whether there is a will or not. Your creditors get whatever assets you had, and your heirs do not have to repay any of your debts or outstanding bills.

LIVING WILL (HEALTH-CARE PROXY)

A "living will," "health-care proxy," and "durable power of attorney for health care" are similar legal documents that can work together to help ensure that your wishes will be carried out regarding your health care and medical treatment, particularly your individual choices regarding the later stages of serious illness and end-of-life issues. In the absence of such docu-

Go confidently in the direction of your dreams! Live the life you've imagined. As you simplify your life, the laws of the universe will be simpler; solitude will not be solitude, poverty will not be poverty, nor weakness.

—HENRY DAVID THOREAU

ments, your health-care professional will continue to follow whatever instructions you gave while you were still able to do so, and may need to contact a family member, which may cause delay, confusion, and conflict.

These documents authorize someone you trust to step in and act on your behalf and judge what you would want or what is best for you under the circumstances. Your agent can be any adult, including a family member. However, there are some limitations if you appoint a health-care professional, as they cannot be your agent and your health-care provider at the same time. It's a good idea also to appoint an alternate, if for some reason your primary choice is unavailable.

It's important to choose someone who you trust will follow *your wishes* even if theirs are different from your own. You should discuss your wishes in detail with this person, your family, and your health-care professionals. You may request that your agent consult others; however, your agent's decisions may overrule the wishes of your relatives, hospital policies, or principles of those providing your care. It's important to understand that treatments can never be given to you or stopped if your doctor has reasonable cause to believe that *you object.*

Even after you have signed this form, as long as you are able to make medical and treatment decisions for yourself, you have the right to do so. Your agent only takes over when the doctors have decided that you are unable to do so. You may cancel health-care proxy at any time simply by informing your agent, either orally or in writing.

You can give this agent as much or as little authority as you want, including the right to make decisions to remove or withhold life-sustaining treatment. This agent is required to follow all your written and oral wishes and limitations, although no one is permitted to stop treatments or withhold artificial nu-

A lot of people will also urge you to put some money in a bank, and in fact—within reason—this is very good advice. But don't go overboard. Remember, what you are doing is giving your money to somebody else to hold on to, and I think that it is worth keeping in mind that the businessmen who run banks are so worried about holding on to things that they put little chains on all their pens.

—MISS PIGGY

trition and hydration—even family members—without your specific prior authorization.

Typically, these documents itemize a list of possible circumstances followed by a list of procedures that you do or do not want, for example:

If I should be in an incurable or irreversible mental or physical condition with no reasonable expectation of recovery and unable to communicate my wishes, I direct that:

- all artificial administration of food and water be withheld.

- all comfort care be provided, even if it would also have the effect of prolonging my life.

- all additional life-prolonging treatment be withheld, including: blood and blood products, cardiopulmonary resuscitation (CPR), diagnostic tests, dialysis, drugs, respirator, and surgery.

- all other therapies and treatments that merely prolong my dying be withheld or withdrawn.

In addition, you can grant your agent the authority to:

- hire and fire medical personnel.

- visit you in a hospital or other medical care facility.

- review and receive any information regarding your physical or mental health, including medical and hospital records.

- sign any releases or other documents required to obtain this information.

- sign any documents required to request,

withdraw, or refuse medical treatment or
to be released or transferred from a hosital
or other medical facility.

+ sign any waiver or release from liability
required by a hospital or physician.

LETTING GO

Living with HIV/AIDS or any other life-challenging disease is about not giving up or giving in, it's about
holding on—one day at a time, if necessary—and doing whatever it takes. But there can come a time when
the body has broken down beyond all reasonable hope
of repair, when there is constant pain, with little expectation of anything beyond more treatments, more
drugs, more hospital visits, and more pain.

*As a well-spent day
brings happy sleep,
so life well used
brings happy death.*
*—LEONARDO
DA VINCI*

Probably the single most difficult decision is
knowing when to stop fighting—when to let go. It's
when you have crossed over the line from being truly
alive to merely existing thanks to medical technology.
It's when you are at peace, and for you, the thought
of death just isn't that scary anymore.

The problem has become so much more difficult
because medical technology has advanced to the point
where the very boundaries between birth, life, and
death have become blurred. The body can be kept
"alive"—in some sense of the word—for long after
what most people would consider death.

With all that *can be done*, the question is what
should be done. The choices that doctors and hospitals
make are sometimes not necessarily the right ones. I
have seen people who still have a lot of fight left in
them written off as being "terminal" and the medical
professionals simply stop trying. This all too often
happens with the elderly and with people with AIDS.

EUTHANASIA, SUICIDE, AND A RIGHT TO DIE

The *Merriam-Webster's Collegiate Dictionary* defines euthanasia as "the act or practice of killing [active euthanasia] or permitting the death [passive euthanasia] of a hopelessly sick or injured individual in a relatively painless way for reasons of mercy."

An example of *passive euthanasia* would be allowing a person in the very advanced stages of AIDS who is in chronic pain to discontinue life-prolonging treatment and discharge him- or herself from the hospital so they may die naturally in the comfort of home or in the comfort of a hospice.

An example of *active euthanasia* would be to administer a lethal injection to that same person to hasten the inevitable end of his or her life and thus reduce his or her suffering.

An example of *physician assisted suicide* would be for a doctor to prescribe drugs and council that same person so that this terminally ill person could end his own life with some quality of life and human dignity.

The whole issue of euthanasia, suicide, and a right to die is very similar to the abortion issue. Most people feel very strongly one way or another about it, and, unfortunately, otherwise rational, intelligent people reach different conclusions, and both sides find the opposing viewpoint both immoral and unacceptable.

At one extreme, there is the belief that all human life must always be preserved by any means possible. "Human life" for some is defined as beginning when the sperm impregnates the ovum and continues until the last signs of life leave the body. For these people, abortion, euthanasia, and suicide are the equivalent of murder and are therefore never an acceptable choice.

At the other extreme is the belief that it is the quality of life that counts, and that there may be times—perhaps only under extreme circumstances—

Eternal truth will be neither true nor eternal unless they have fresh meaning for every new social situation.
—FRANKLIN D.
ROOSEVELT

when abortion, euthanasia, or suicide may be the most appropriate, humane, and moral choice.

Like all other ethical, moral, spiritual, and religious questions, each person must find the answers for his own situation within himself. Of course, since no one may impose their choices on others, those that are directly affected, and *only* those that are directly affected—the people, families, friends, religious groups, or the community as a whole—must similarly search inside to find what's right. Outsiders may help us along the way, in the end it is a personal journey.

Regardless of what your personal views on these issues are, it is important to be clear on them, express your beliefs to your immediate friends and family. For information on this subject, refer to some of the books in "Appendix A: Suggested Reading," the section on *The Practical Side of Death, Dying, and Grief,* or contact a national advocacy organization such as Choice in Dying or The Hemlock Society (see "Appendix B: National and Regional Resources").

HELPFUL HINTS AFTER A DEATH

When someone dies, there are all sorts of practical things that need to be taken care of *right away* and most of us, luckily, don't have a lot of experience with this sort of thing. To make matters worse, the very people who need to make all these important decisions and take these actions are not at their best, nor are they thinking very objectively.

This is why a little advance planning can help so much, and having the guideline of a document stating exactly what someone would have wanted makes the process just that much easier.

Although the final decision rests with your personal representative (executor) or heirs, documenting your final wishes helps them know what you would have wanted. Of course, you can't know the exact circumstances that your folks will have to work with

[Alice asked]
"Would you tell me, please, which way I ought to go from here?"

"That depends a good deal on where you want to get to," said the [Cheshire] Cat.

"I don't much care where—" said Alice.

"Then it doesn't matter which way you go," said the Cat.

"—so long as I get somewhere," Alice added as an explanation.

"Oh you're sure to do that," said the Cat, *"if only you walk long enough."*
—LEWIS CAROLL
Alice in Wonderland

after you die, so encourage your personal representative (executor) or heirs to make whatever adjustments are appropriate to make things as easy and comforting for everyone as possible.

When I was in high school, one of my classes entailed a required field trip to a funeral home. The idea was that sometime in our lives—probably many years into the future—we would have to make arrangements for the funeral of a loved one, and that it would be so much easier if we had gone through a dry run.

For us, it was almost a joke, so we asked all sorts of questions—the way all teenagers do—that we wouldn't dream of asking if one of our parents, children, siblings, or spouse was lying dead in the next room. We were encouraged to ask all sorts of ghoulish questions that would have been considered normal and practical if it had been any other topic. We learned how much things cost and what choices were fashionable with what group of customers. We learned that the funeral home was like a caterer or travel agent who coordinated all the details, arrangements, and vendors.

Our homework was to write a detailed plan and budget for some dearly departed imaginary relative. We were strongly encouraged to discuss this with the rest of our family to see how they would feel about it. A lot of students and families were shocked by this assignment, but for me it was a good opportunity to talk with my parents about a subject that otherwise we might never have brought up.

For our project, most of us either planned a $50,000 production suitable for a Hollywood superstar, or we chose the $500 no-frills cremation option. Real funerals don't work that way. As we've said earlier in this chapter, funerals and memorials are for the living, so you need to think about the needs of those

A heathen came before Shammai and said to him, "take me as a proselyte, but on condition that you teach me the entire torah, all of it, while I stand on one foot." Shammai instantly drove him away. When the heathen came before Hillel, Hillel said to him "love thy neighbor as thyself. This is the entire torah, all of it: the rest is commentary. Now go and study it."

—MISHNA

who will attend and participate in this process. Local laws and customs also may dictate what is possible. The important thing is to mix and match to select whatever options will help these people the most:

- type of casket (no-frills/wood/sealed metal)

- wake (open/closed casket/none)

- body embalmed/not

- funerals or precremation/preburial ceremony (religious/nonreligious/none)

- send flowers/donate to charity

- cremation (scatter ashes/inter ashes)

- burial (aboveground/in-ground vault/in-ground/none)

- gravestone/marker/memorial/none

- memorial service/celebration of life/none or postcremation/postburial ceremony

- When: funerals are anywhere from the next day to within a week. Memorials are sometimes a month or more away. Be careful not to delay things too long; most people need some event to cope with the initial grieving process.

There are people who have money and people who are rich.
—COCO GABRIELLE CHANEL

Once the arrangements have been coordinated with the funeral home, then comes the important task of passing along this information to everyone who might need to know. This usually involves working through the deceased's address book and making dozens of phone calls. Although this sounds like a lot of work, quite frankly, it's often nice to have something practical to do at this time.

Purchase a new address book. Recopy, update (or delete), and organize all the names, addresses, and phone numbers into a single book. Are there other names and phone numbers you have memorized? Add these too. Neatness and completeness count. Remember, you might not be the only person who has to use it. I like to go through this process every Thanksgiving in preparation for sending Christmas cards.

You might also consider placing a memorial advertisement in with the local AIDS services organization newsletter. It's a good way to show support, and to notify more casual friends and HIV/AIDS support buddies.

Shop around for the right funeral home, preferably well in advance of your needs. Make sure that you feel comfortable with them, and that they have some experience in working with people with your special needs and cultural traditions.

Discuss the HIV/AIDS issue, your religion, language, ethnic background, people with special needs, and perhaps even your sexual preference. A number of years ago, many funeral homes refused to work with people who had HIV/AIDS and felt uncomfortable with openly gay people. Thankfully, because of a general enlightenment in the industry, today there is rarely a problem, even outside of the big cities. But just in case, it's better to find out beforehand, while you can choose an alternative, rather than at the last minute.

Often the funeral home, the newspapers, friends, and family will all ask if there is a nice photograph of the deceased. Too often, one has to do without, or use an antique from the high school yearbook. Perhaps I'm just too vain or grandiose, but I wanted to make sure that I would look good, so this was an added incentive to get a flattering photo studio portrait. Besides it makes such a lovely Christmas gift.

One of the situations in which everybody seems to fear loneliness is death. In tones drenched with pity, people say of someone, "He died alone." I have never understood this point of view. Who wants to have to die and be polite at the same time?

—QUENTIN CRISP

SKELETONS IN THE CLOSET

It's not only elected officials that have a few skeletons in the closets. Most of us have something personal, private, or embarrassing: old love letters, private diaries and photographs, memorabilia from some phase of our past, pornography, sex toys, drugs, or the assorted paraphernalia of some secret vice, all sorts of things that we would rather others didn't see.

Death doesn't always come according to our schedule, and sometimes people die unexpectedly. Too often I have seen a grieving parent, grandparent, or child learn much more about their loved one than they ever wanted to know.

The best advice, by far, is if you don't want others to see these things later on, get rid of them yourself before you die. Another alternative is to make an agreement with a best friend to dispose of things for you, and vice versa.

If no arrangements of this sort have been made, as a good friend of someone who just died, you might consider giving his or her home the once-over. If you do find anything that your friend might have felt uncomfortable about, you can always ask the family what they would like to do with these "very personal, private things that so-and-so would have wished kept private." Be very careful about this, because sometimes, it is just these clues that a grieving loved one needs to piece together a life that they didn't have the opportunity to share.

When all this is over, then comes the time for the personal representative (executor) who was appointed in the will to go through all the bureaucratic nightmares of settling the estate in probate court in the deceased's legal state of residence at the time of his or her death, *as listed on the death certificate.*

At best, this is never easy and will require the assistance of some legal counseling. Being organized and keeping careful notes will help a lot. You will also

The ultimate measure of a man is not where he stands in moments of comfort and convenience, but where he stands at times of challenge and controversy.
—MARTIN LUTHER KING, JR.

need somewhere between four and twenty-four—with about eight being normal—official copies of the death certificate to send to anyone who holds an asset, such as a bank, or anyone who is owed money, such as a hospital.

GETTING ON WITH LIFE

Finally, after all the paperwork is complete, and the estate is finally closed, there comes the very long process for those left behind to get on with their lives, to carry their love with them in their hearts, let go of the past, and begin reinventing their future.

This, of course, brings us right back to Chapter 1 . . .

I have a right to my anger, and I don't want anybody telling me I shouldn't be, that it's not nice to be, and that something's wrong with me because I get angry.

—MAXINE WATERS

SUGGESTED READING

In keeping with this book's theme that each person must find what is right for him- or herself, what follows are some suggestions, options, and directions to go from here to get more information.

Personally, I'm an information junkie. The more information, the better. But choosing the most useful resources isn't easy. There are literally thousands and thousands of HIV/AIDS-related books. Tens of thousands more if you include all the general self-help, health, fitness, medical reference, recovery, gay/lesbian, women's/men's, motivational, inspirational, psychology, philosophy, religious, and spiritual books as well. Many of these are either too technically specific, too general, or too outdated to be of much use.

Such a large selection can be overwhelming. In "Appendix A," I've selected about 150 of what I feel are the best books grouped into twenty-one general categories. Some people will be initially scared off by such a long list. Don't be. It's intended to be used like a menu at a restaurant: giving you lots of choices and suggestions, but you aren't supposed to pick too much at any one sitting . This is *not* a required reading list.

In each category there are a number of viewpoints and styles. Within each category, books are listed roughly according to the order that you might want to consider reading them. This order is purely subjective, and is based on the book's ease of use,

There is one thing stronger than all the armies of the world, and that is an idea whose time has come.

—VICTOR HUGO

The way a book is read—which is to say, the qualities a reader brings to a book—can have as much to do with its worth as anything the author puts into it.

—NORMAN COUSINS

availability, cost, as well as its content and style. Each of you should be able to find at least one or two books in each category that meet your unique needs.

There are also countless other books and resources that can be invaluable as well. Finding them can be something of a challenge in itself. When faced with anything new—anything from trying to figure out how to write and sell a book such as this, how to survive bicycling hundred of miles, or how to survive and thrive with HIV/AIDS—I love to "go digging" and find out as much as I can in as short a period of time as I can.

A great place to start is by contacting some of the organizations in "Appendix B: National and Regional Resources" and see what books, magazines, publications, and workshops they have to offer you. You will probably want to go to a good library or bookstore and browse through one of those huge magazine sections and see what's out there. If you have access to a computer and a modem (and a few bucks to spend), dial into America Online and almost every other computer service, bulletin boards, or internet host you can find. See what resources recommend other resources.

Once you have all this information sitting in front of you, it's not always easy to tell what information resources will be helpful, and which ones are useless, or even harmful. It's a good idea to consider the source and age of the information as well as what others you know of think about this resource. You might want to consider:

Date of publication: Information about HIV/AIDS changes quickly. For HIV/AIDS-specific titles, anything older than three or four years is probably too old.

Author: Who is this person? Have you heard good things about his or her other works? Does the author have the experience and/or credentials to offer sound information?

"Classic"—A Book which people praise and don't read.
—MARK TWAIN

Endorsements: Have other authors, experts, and organizations that you know and trust agreed with or endorsed this work, or referred to it in their books and publications? Is this sponsored by some organization that has some interest in selling you something?

When you find something worthwhile, share it, particularly at support groups and AIDS services organizations. I'm always updating and improving this list of information resources. If you find a particularly good resource that isn't here, or have a bad experience with one that is, please drop me a note at the address on the page at the back of the book. Happy hunting!

LIST OF CATEGORIES

+ A Beginning
+ What Is Healing?
+ Becoming an HIV/AIDS Expert
+ Medical Self-Empowerment
+ Personal Self-Empowerment
+ People's Inspiring Stories
+ Special Interest for Women
+ Holistic Treatment and Nutritional Therapy
+ Philosophy and Spirituality
+ Finding Your Life's Purpose
+ Addiction and Recovery
+ Meditation and Daily Thoughts
+ Stress Reduction and Exercise
+ Sexuality
+ Educating Others
+ Helping Others
+ Directories

I came to the conclusion that one of the reasons why I'm so blessed, I think, is because I reach so many people, and you never know whose life you are touching or affecting. And so, because your blessings come back to you based upon how you give them out . . . that's why I'm so . . . You know what I'm saying? You get it? OK, good.

—OPRAH WINFREY

- The Practical Side of Death, Dying, and Grief
- The Emotional Side of Death, Dying, and Grieving
- Politics/History
- Miscellaneous

A BEGINNING

Living Positively in a World with HIV/AIDS
by Mark de Solla Price
1995; 288 pages; $10.00; Avon Books
ISBN: 0-380-77623-5

You Can't Afford the Luxury of a Negative Thought: A Book for People with Any Life-Threatening Illness—Including Life
by John-Roger and Peter McWilliams
1988; 622 pages; $14.95; Prelude Press
ISBN: 0-931580-20-X

Love, Medicine, and Miracles: Lessons Learned about Self-Healing from a Surgeon's Experience with Exceptional Patients
by Bernie S. Siegel
1990; 256 pages; $12.00; HarperCollins
ISBN: 0-06-091983-3

Quantum Healing: Exploring the Frontiers of Body, Mind, Medicine
by Depak Chopra
1990; $10.00; Bantam Books
ISBN: 0-553-34869-8

Anatomy of an Illness As Perceived by the Patient
by Norman Cousins
1991; 176 pages; $10.00; Bantam Books
ISBN: 0-553-35481-7

You Can Heal Your Life
by Louise Hay
1987; 240 pages; $12.00; Hay House
ISBN: 0-937611-01-8

Type A Behavior and Your Heart
by Meyer Friedman and Ray Rosenman
1974; 319 pages; $4.95; Fawcett Books
ISBN: 0-449-20073-6

The Power of Positive Thinking
by Norman Vincent Peale
1992; $5.95; Fawcett Books
ISBN: 0-449-45093-7

Who Gets Sick: How Beliefs, Moods, and Thoughts Affect Your Health
by Blair Justice, Ph.S.
1987; 327 pages; $13.95; Jeremy P. Tarcher, Inc./St. Martin's Press
ISBN: 0-87477-507-8

WHAT IS HEALING?

The Heart of Healing
by The Institute of Noetic Sciences with William Poole
1993; 192 pages; $24.95; Turner Publishing
ISBN: 1-878685-44-9

Healing and the Mind
by Bill Moyers
1993; 369 pages; Bantam Doubleday Dell
ISBN: 0-385-46870-9

The Wellness Encyclopedia: The Comprehensive Family Resource
from the editors of the University of California, Berkeley Wellness Letter

1992; 541 pages; $15.45; Houghton
  Mifflin
ISBN: 0-395-61330-2

Wellness Workbook, Second Edition
by John W. Travis, M.D. and Regina Sara
  Ryan
1988; 238 pages; $13.95; Ten Speed Press
ISBN: 0-89815-179-1

*The Secret of Life: Redesigning the Living
World*
by Joseph Levine and David Suzuki
(Companion to the PBS Television Series)
1993; 280 pages; $24.95; WGBH Boston
ISBN: 0-9636881-0-3

BECOMING AN HIV/AIDS EXPERT

*The Guide to Living with HIV Infection:
Developed at the Johns Hopkins AIDS Clinic,
Revised Edition*
by John G. Bartlett and Ann K.
  Finkbeiner
1993; 359 pages; $15.95; Johns Hopkins
  University Press
ISBN: 0-8018-4664-1

*No Time To Wait: A Complete Guide to
Treating, Managing, and Living with HIV
Infection*
by Nick Siano with Suzanne Lipsett
1993; 367 pages; $12.95; Bantam Books
ISBN: 0-553-37176-2

Early Care for HIV Disease, Second Edition
by Ronald A. Baker, Jeffrey M. Moulton,
  John Tighe
1992; 144 pages; San Francisco AIDS
  Foundation
(Available from "Impact AIDS" at
  [415] 861-3397)
no ISBN

The Essential AIDS Fact Book
by Paul Harding Douglas and Laura
  Pinsky/Columbia University Health
  Service
1992; 108 pages; $7.50; Pocket Books
ISBN: 0-671-73184-X

*The HIV Test: What You Need to Know to
Make an Informed Decision*
by Marc E. Vargo, M.S.
1992; $9.00; Pocket Books
ISBN: 0-671-77950-8

*STD: Sexually Transmitted Diseases,
Including HIV/AIDS*
by John T. Daugirdas, M.D.
1992; 150 pages; $9.00; Medtext
  (708-325-3277)
ISBN: 0-9629279-1-0

The Science of AIDS
edited by *Scientific American Magazine*
1989; 135 pages; $12.95; W. H. Freeman
ISBN: 0-7167-2036-1

AIDS: Problems and Prospects
by Lawrence Corey, M.D., editor
162 pages; $19.95; HP Publishing
(rather technical, from *Hospital Practice
  Magazine*)
ISBN: 0-393-71015-7

*Immune Power: A Comprehensive Healing
Program for HIV*
by Jon D. Kaiser, M.D.
1993; 192 pages; $18.95; St. Martin's
  Press
ISBN: 0-312-09312-8

Living with AIDS: Reaching Out
by Tom O'Connor with Ahmed
  Gonzalez-Nunez

1986; 375 pages; $18.95; Corwin
Publishers
ISBN: 0-938569-00-7

HIV + : Working the System
by Robert A. Rimer and Michael A.
Connolly
1993; 236 pages; $12.95; Alyson
Publications
ISBN: 1-55583-208-3

Understanding and Preventing AIDS: A Book
for Everyone, Second Edition
by Chris Jennings
1988; 240 pages; $24.95; Health Alert
Press
ISBN: 0-936571-01-2

Pathways to Wellness: Strategies for
Self-Empowerment in the Age of AIDS
by Paul Kent Froman
1990; 282 pages; $10.95; Penguin/Plume
ISBN: 0-452-26437-5

Understanding the Basics: An Overview
of HIV
[audiotape]
by Brian N. Kleis, M.D.
1994; $4.95; Life Management
This and many more HIV/AIDS audiotapes
are available by calling (800) 635-3379.

MEDICAL SELF-EMPOWERMENT

How to Live Between Office Visits: A Guide
to Life, Love and Healing
by Bernie S. Siegel
1993; 256 pages; $22.00; HarperCollins
ISBN: 0-06-016800-5

AIDS and the Healer Within, Updated Edition
by Nick Bamforth
1993; 172 pages; $9.95; Amethyst Books
ISBN: 0-944256-27-9

Take Charge of Your Health: Professional
Secrets You Need to Know to Obtain the Best
Medical Care
by Stephen Astor, M.D.
1991; 205 pages; Two A's Industries, Inc.
ISBN: 0-915001-07-1

Peace, Love and Healing: Bodymind
Communication and the Path to Self-Healing:
An Exploration
by Bernie S. Siegel
1990; 293 pages; $12.00; HarperCollins
ISBN: 0-06-091705-9

Perfect Health: The Complete Mind-Body
Guide
by Depak Chopra
1991; 336 pages; $12.00; Crown
Publishing
ISBN: 0-517-58421-2

Creating Health: How to Wake up the Body's
Intelligence
by Depak Chopra
1991; 234 pages; $8.70; Houghton Mifflin
ISBN: 0-395-57421-8

Head First: The Biology of Hope and the
Healing Power of the Human Spirit
by Norman Cousins
1990; 380 pages; $9.95; Viking Penguin
ISBN: 0-14-013965-6

Be Sick Well: A Healthy Approach to Chronic
Illness
by Jeff Kane, M.D.
1991; 188 pages; $11.95; New Harbinger
Publications
ISBN: 1-879237-08-3

Meeting the Challenge of Disability or Chronic
Illness: A Family Guide
by Lori Goldfarb, et. al.

1986; 210 pages; Paul H. Brookes
Publishing Company
ISBN: 0-933716-55-9

PERSONAL
SELF-EMPOWERMENT

*Man with No Name: How the Founder of the
Famous Amos Cookie Company Lost
Everything, Including His Name—and
Turned Adversity into Opportunity*
by Wally Amos
1994; 154 pages; $9.95; Aslan Publishing
ISBN: 0-944031-57-9

Love Is Letting Go of Fear
by Gerald Jampolsky
1988; 144 pages; $7.95; Celestial Arts
ISBN: 0-89087-246-5

*LIFE 101: Everything We Wish We Had
Learned about Life in School—but Didn't*
by Peter and John-Roger McWilliams
1991; 399 pages; $11.95; Prelude Press
ISBN: 0-931580-97-8

Healing the Shame That Binds You
by John Bradshaw
1988; $9.95; Health Communications
ISBN: 0-932194-86-9

*Homecoming: Reclaiming and Championing
Your Inner Child*
by John Bradshaw
1992; 304 pages; $12.50; Bantam Books
ISBN: 0-553-35389-6

Do It!: Let's Get off Our Butts
by Peter and John-Roger McWilliams
1992; 496 pages; $11.95; Prelude Press
ISBN: 0-931580-96-X

PEOPLE'S INSPIRING STORIES

Living Proof
[a beautiful photographic essay of people
living with HIV/AIDS]
by Carolyn Jones
1994; Abbeville Press
ISBN: 1-55859-7131

Beyond AIDS: A Journey into Healing
by George R. Melton with Wil Garcia
1988; 168 pages; $10.00; Brotherhood
Press
ISBN: 0-9621959-0-1

Surviving AIDS
by Michael Callen
1991 (originally 1990); 256 pages;
$10.00; HarperCollins
ISBN: 0-06-092125-0

They Conquered AIDS!: True Life Adventures
by Scott J. Gregory and Bianca Leonardo
1989; 360 pages; $19.95; Tree of Life
ISBN: 0-930852-03-6

Why I Survive AIDS
by Niro Markoff and Paul Duffy
1991; 288 pages; $10.00; Simon &
Schuster/Fireside
ISBN: 0-671-68352-7

My Own Story
by Ryan White and Ann Marie
Cunningham
1992; 326 pages; $4.95; Signet
ISBN: 0-451-17322-8

Borrowed Time: An AIDS Memoir
by Paul Monette
1990; $9.95; Avon Books
ISBN: 0-3807-0779-9

Someone You Know: A Friend's Farewell
by Maria Pallotta-Chiarolli
1991; 188 pages; Wakefield Press
ISBN: 1-86254-271-6

Roger's Recovery from AIDS
by Bob L. Owen
1992 (originally 1987); 214 pages; Health
    Digest
ISBN: 1-882657-00-4

Voices That Care: Stories and Encouragements
for People with HIV/AIDS and Those Who
Love Them
by Neal Hitchens
1992; 271 pages; $11.00; Fireside/Simon
    & Schuster
ISBN: 0-671-88230-9

AIDS Stories of Living Longer
edited by C. Ray
1991; 32 pages; $3.25; Taterhill Press
ISBN: 0-9616792-9-8

My Own Country: A Doctor's Story of a
Town and Its People in the Age of AIDS
by Abraham Verghese
1994; 347 pages; $23.00; Simon &
    Schuster
ISBN: 0-671-78514-1

SPECIAL INTEREST FOR WOMEN

A Shallow Pool of Time: One HIV-positive
Woman Grapples with the AIDS Epidemic
by Fran Peavey
1990; 268 pages; $12.95; New Society
    Publishers
ISBN: 0-86571-167-4

Women and HIV/AIDS: An International
Resource Book
by Marge Berer with Sunanda Ray

1993; 383 pages; $22.00; Pandora Press/
    HarperCollins
ISBN: 0-04-440876-5

Positive Women: Voices of Women Living
with AIDS
edited by Andrea Rudd and Darien Taylor
1992; 269 pages; $14.95; Second Story
    Press/Inbook
ISBN: 0-929005-30-9

The Invisible Epidemic: The Story of Women
and AIDS
by Gena Corea
1993; 356 pages; $12.00; Harper
    Perennial
ISBN: 0-06-092191

Our Bodies, Ourselves, Second Edition,
Revised
The Boston Women's Health Book
    Collective Staff
1976; 352 pages; $14.95; Simon &
    Schuster
ISBN: 0-671-22145-0

Women, AIDS, and Activism
by ACT-UP—New York Women and
    AIDS Book Group
1990; 295 pages; $9.00; South End Press
ISBN: 0-89608-393-4

HOLISTIC TREATMENT AND NUTRITIONAL THERAPY

HIV+ Survival Guide: Diet for Living in the
Age of HIV/AIDS
[videotape]
1994; $39.95; Lifeforce
This videotape is available by calling
    (800) 788-8823.

Treating AIDS with Chinese Medicine
by Mary Kay Ryan and Arthur D. Shattuck
1994; 361 pages; $29.95; Pacific View Press
ISBN: 1-881896-07-2

Nine Ounces: A Nine Part Program for the Prevention of AIDS In HIV-Positive Persons [with Chinese Medicine]
by Bob Flaws
1992; 84 pages; $9.95; Blue Poppy Press
ISBN: 0-936185-12-0

A Holistic Protocol for the Immune System: A Manual for HIV-ARC-AIDS and Other Opportunistic Infections, Fifth Edition
by Scott J. Gregory and Bianca Leonardo
1993; 120 pages; $15.95; Tree of Life
ISBN: 0-930852-22-2

Healing AIDS Naturally: Natural Therapies for the Immune System
by Laurence E. Badgley
1987; 410 pages; $14.95; Human Energy Press
ISBN: 0-941523-00-4

Surviving with AIDS: A Comprehensive Program of Nutritional Co-Therapy
by C. Wayne Callaway and Catherine Whitney
1991; 192 pages; $14.95; Little, Brown and Company
ISBN: 0-3161-2467-2

Natural Immunity: Insights on Diet and AIDS
by Noboru B. Muramoto
1988; 323 pages; $12.95; George Ohsawa Macrobiotic Foundation
ISBN: 0-918860-48-2

Nutrition and HIV/AIDS: Practical Steps for a Healthier Life
by Gustavo Wong, RD
1993; 21 pages; Physicians Association for AIDS Care
To order call (800) 238-7828.

AIDS, Macrobiotics, and Natural Immunity
by Michio Kushi, Martha C. Cottrell, Mark N. Mead
1990; 496 pages; $19.95; Japan Publications
ISBN: 0-87040-680-9

Creative Choices Cookbook: A Minimax™ Book
by Graham Kerr
1993; 209 pages; $21.95; G.P. Putnam's Sons
ISBN: 0-399-13896-X

Beyond Pritikin: A Total Nutrition Program...for Longevity and Good Health
by Ann L. Gittleman and John M. Desgrey
1989; 240 pages; $5.99; Bantam Books
ISBN: 0-553-27512-7

The Corinne T. Netzer Encyclopedia of Food Values
by Corinne T. Netzer
1992; 903 pages; $25.00; Dell Publishing
ISBN: 0-440-50367-1

PHILOSOPHY AND SPIRITUALITY

A Return to Love: Reflections on the Principles of a Course in Miracles
by Marianne Williamson
1992; 320 pages; $12.00; HarperCollins
ISBN: 0-06-092341-5

The Tibetan Book of Living and Dying
by Sogyal Rinpoche

1992; 425 pages; $22.00; Harper San
Francisco
ISBN: 0-06-250793-1

The Tao of Pooh
by Benjamin Hoff
1983; 158 pages; $9.00; Viking/Penguin
ISBN: 0-14-006747-7

*All I Really Need to Know I Learned in
Kindergarten: Uncommon Thoughts on
Common Things*
by Robert Fulghum
1991; 208 pages; $5.95; Ballantine/Ivy
Books
ISBN: 0-8041-0526-X

A Course in Miracles, Second Revised Edition
edited by Helen Schucman
1992; 1,296 pages; $25.00; Foundation for
Inner Peace
ISBN: 0-9606388-8-1

Living in the Light
by Shakti Gawain and Laurel King
1986; 220 pages; $9.95; New World
Library
ISBN: 0-931432-14-6

*For Those We Love: A Spiritual Perspective
on AIDS, Second Edition*
by Catholic Archdiocese of St. Paul and
Minneapolis, AIDS Ministry Program
Staff
with illustrations by Jim Debruycker
1991; 112 pages; $8.95; Pilgrim Press/
United Church Press
ISBN: 0-8298-0919-8

*Emmanuel's Book: A Manual for Living
Comfortably in the Cosmos*
by Pat Rodegast and Judith Stanton
1985; $10.00; Bantam Books
ISBN: 0-9615090-0-7

Emmanuel's Book II: The Choice for Love
by Pat Rodegast and Judith Stanton
1989; $9.95; Bantam Books
ISBN: 0-553-34750-0

I Come As a Brother
by Bartholomew (M. Moore)
1986; 175 pages; $10.95; High Mesa
Press
ISBN: 0-9614010-0-1

*Chop Wood, Carry Water: A Guide to
Finding Spiritual Fulfillment in Everyday Life*
by Rick Fields, Peggy Taylor, Rex Weyler,
and Rick Ingrasci and the editors of
New Age Journal
1984; 304 pages; $13.95; Jeremy P.
Tarcher
ISBN: 0-87477-209-5

*As Above, So Below: Paths to Spiritual
Renewal in Daily Life*
by Ronald S. Miller and the editors of *New
Age Journal*
1992; 346 pages; $13.95; Jeremy P.
Tarcher
ISBN: 0-87477-659-7

*Road Less Traveled: A New Psychology of
Love, Traditional Values and Spiritual
Growth*
by M. Scott Peck
1988; 320 pages; $13.00; Simon &
Schuster/Touchstone
ISBN: 0-671-67300-9

*The Different Drum: Community Making and
Peace*
by M. Scott Peck
1988; 336 pages; $10.00; Simon &
Schuster/Touchstone
ISBN: 0-671-66833-1

FINDING YOUR LIFE'S PURPOSE

*The 1995 What Color Is Your Parachute?:
A Practical Manual for Job Hunters and
Career Changers*
by Richard Nelson Bolles
1994; 480 pages; $14.95; Ten Speed Press
ISBN: 0-89815-633-5

*Please Understand Me: Character and
Temperament Types*
by David Keirsey and Marilyn Bates
1984; 209 pages; $11.95; Prometheus
   Nemesis Books
ISBN: 0-9606954-0-0

*Type Talk: The 16 Personality Types That
Determine How We Live, Love, and Work*
by Otto Kroeger and Janet M. Thuesen
1988; 193 pages; $9.95; Tilden Press
   Books
ISBN: 0-385-29828-5

*WEALTH 101: Getting What You Want—
Enjoying What You've Got*
by Peter and John-Roger McWilliams
1992; 532 pages; $19.95; Prelude Press
ISBN: 0-931580-50-1

*The Secrets of Consulting: A Guide to Giving
and Getting Advice Successfully*
by Gerald M. Weinberg, forward by
   Virginia Satir
1985; 248 pages; $28.00; Dorset House
ISBN: 0-932633-01-3

Getting Things Done
by Edwin C. Bliss
1984; $4.95; Bantam Books
ISBN: 0-553-27384-1

Doing It Now
by Edwin C. Bliss

1984; 224 pages; $3.95; Bantam Books
ISBN: 0-553-26017-0

ADDICTION AND RECOVERY

Living Sober
1975; 87 pages; $1.20; Alcoholics
   Anonymous
ISBN: 0-916856-04-6

Narcotics Anonymous
1988; 286 pages; Narcotics Anonymous
ISBN: 1-55776-025-X

*Circle of Hope: Our Stories of AIDS, Addiction
and Recovery*
by Perry Tilleraas
1990; 364 pages; $11.00; Hazelden
   Education Materials
ISBN: 0-89486-610-9

*The Alternative Twelve Steps: A Secular
Guide to Recovery*
by Martha Cleveland and Arlys G.
   Cleveland
1992; 136 pages; $8.95; Health
   Communications
ISBN: 1-55874-167-4

MEDITATION AND DAILY
THOUGHTS

*The Color of Light: Meditations for All of Us
Living with AIDS*
by Perry Tilleraas
1988; 400 pages; $9.00; Hazelden
   Educational Materials
ISBN: 0-89486-511-0

*The Tao of Healing: Meditations for Body and
Spirit*
by Haven Trevino; preface by Gerald
   Jampolsky
1993; 96 pages; $9.95; New World
   Library
ISBN: 1-880032-18-X

Meditations from the Road
by M. Scott Peck
1993; 384 pages; $9.00; Simon &
Schuster
ISBN: 0-671-79799-9

*Reflections in the Light: Daily Thoughts and
Meditations*
by Shakti Gawain
1988; 400 pages; $9.95; New World
Library
ISBN: 0-931432-13-8

*365 Tao: Daily Meditations by Deng
Ming-Dao*
1992; 380 pages; $12.00; HarperCollins
ISBN: 0-06-250223-9

STRESS REDUCTION AND EXERCISE

Stretching
by Bob Anderson
1986; 192 pages; $9.95; Random House
ISBN: 0-394-73874-8

*Kicking Your Stress Habits: A Do-It-Yourself
Guide for Coping with Stress*
by Donald A. Tubesing
1991; 187 pages; $14.95; Whole Person
Associates
ISBN: 0-938586-00-9

*Relax, Recover: Stress Management for
Recovering People*
by Patricia Wuertzer and Lucinda May
1988; 140 pages; Hazelden Educational
Materials
ISBN: 0-89486-495-5

SEXUALITY

*The Advocate Adviser [of gay issues and
sexuality]*
by Pat Califia

1991; 237 pages; $8.95; Alyson
Publications
ISBN: 1-55583-169-9

Safer Sex: The Guide to Gay Sex Safely
by Peter Tatchell, photographs by Robert
Taylor
1994; 128 pages; $19.95; Cassell
ISBN: 0-304-32845-6

The Wonderful Little Sex Book
by William Ashoka Ross
1992; 288 pages; $9.95; Conari Press
ISBN: 0-943233-34-8

*Making It: A Woman's Guide to Sex in the
Age of AIDS*
by Cindy Patton and Janis Kelly
1990; 56 pages; $4.95; Firebrand Books
ISBN: 0-932379-32-X

*Anal Pleasure and Health: A Guide for Men
and Women, Second Edition*
by Jack Morin, Ph.D.
1986; 269 pages; $12.50; Yes Press
ISBN: 0-940208-08-3

EDUCATING OTHERS

*Risky Times: How to Be AIDS-Smart and Stay
Healthy: A Guide for Teenagers*
by Jeanne Blake
1990; 196 pages; $5.95; Workman
Publishing
ISBN: 0-89480-656-4

Fifty Things You Can Do about AIDS
by Neal Hitchens
1992; 96 pages; $6.95; Lowell House
ISBN: 0-929923-95-2

What You Can Do to Avoid AIDS
by Earvin "Magic" Johnson

1992; 192 pages; $3.99; Random House
ISBN: 0-8129-2063-5

HELPING OTHERS

We Are All Living with AIDS: How You Can Set Policies and Guidelines for the Workplace
by Earl C. Pike
1993; 396 pages; $14.95; Deaconess Press
ISBN: 0-925190-68-3

The AIDS Caregiver's Handbook
edited by Ted Eidson
1993; 364 pages; $14.95; St. Martin's Press
ISBN: 0-312-08129-4

Caring for a Loved One with AIDS: The Experiences of Families, Lovers, and Friends
by Marie Annette Brown and Gail M. Powell-Cape
1992; 61 pages; $4.95; University of Washington Press
ISBN: 0-295-97183-5

Among Friends: Hospice Care for the Person with HIV/AIDS
by Robert W. Buckingham
1992; 191 pages; $13.95; Prometheus Books
ISBN: 0-87975-759-0

DIRECTORIES

Local AIDS Services: The National Directory
March 1994; 266 pages; $15; United States Conference of Mayors
(202-293-7300)

How to Find Information About AIDS, Second Edition
edited by Jeffrey T. Huber
1991; 302 pages; $19.95; Haworth Press
ISBN: 0-918393-99-X

Living with AIDS: A Guide to Resources in New York City, 3rd Edition
from Gay Men's Health Crisis, Inc.
1993; 174 pages; $6.00
To order contact GMHC (212) 807-6655.

THE PRACTICAL SIDE OF DEATH, DYING, AND GRIEF

WillMaker 5 (computer software for Macintosh, Windows, and DOS)
[*Helps you think things through and prepare a legal will, living will (health-care directive), and document your final wishes/arrangements.*]
1994; $69.95; Nolo Press
To order call (800) 992-6656.

Final Celebrations: A Guide for Personal and Family Funeral Planning
by Kathleen Sublette and Martin Flagg
1992; 144 pages; $9.95; Pathfinder
ISBN: 0-934793-43-3

Final Exit [euthanasia]
by Derek Humphry
1992; $10.00; Dell
ISBN: 0-440-50488-0

Lawful Exit [euthanasia]
by Derek Humphry
1993; $9.95; North Lane Press
ISBN: 0-9637280-0-8

How to Survive the Loss of a Love
by Peter McWilliams, Melba Colgrove, and Harold Bloomfield
1991; 200 pages; $10.00; Prelude Press
ISBN: 0-931580-45-5

THE EMOTIONAL SIDE OF DEATH, DYING, AND GRIEVING

Recovering from the Loss of a Loved One to AIDS: Help for Surviving Family, Friends, and Lovers Who Grieve
by Katherine Fair Donnelly
1994; 252 pages; $22.95; St. Martin's Press
ISBN: 0-312-11050-2

On Death and Dying
by Elisabeth Kübler-Ross
1970; 260 pages; $7.95; Macmillan/Collier
ISBN: 0-02-089130-X

Healing into Life and Death
by Stephen Levine
1989; $8.95; Doubleday
ISBN: 0-385-26219-1

Embraced by the Light
by Betty J. Eadie and Curtis Taylor
1992; $14.95; Gold Leaf Press
ISBN: 1-882723-00-7

Who Dies: An Investigation of Conscious Living and Dying
by Stephen Levine
1982; 336 pages; $9.95; Doubleday
ISBN: 0-385-17010-6

After You Say Goodbye: When Someone You Love Dies of AIDS
by Paul Kent Froman, Ph.D.
1992; 270 pages; $10.95; Pathfinder
ISBN: 0-8118-0088-1

A Promise to Remember: The NAMES Project Book of Letters
edited by Joe Brown
1992; 256 pages; $10.00; Avon Books
ISBN: 0-380-76711-2

The Quilt: Stories from The NAMES Project
by Cindy Ruskin
1988; 160 pages; $22.95; Pocket Books
ISBN: 0-671-66597-9

POLITICS/HISTORY

History of AIDS: Emergence and Origin of a Modern Pandemic
by Mirko D. Grmek
1990; 279 pages; Princeton Paperbacks
ISBN: 0-691-02477-4

And the Band Played On: Politics, People, and the AIDS Epidemic
by Randy Shilts
1988; 688 pages; $15.00; Viking/Penguin
ISBN: 0-14-011369-X

The AIDS War: Propaganda, Profiteering, and Genocide from the Medical-Industrial Complex
by John Lauritsen
1992; 400 pages; Pagan Press/Asklepios
ISBN: 0-943742-08-0

Poison by Prescription: The AZT Story
by John Lauritsen
1990; 192 pages; $12.00; Pagan Press/ Asklepios
ISBN: 0-943742-06-4

Bearing Witness: Gay Men's Health Crisis and the Politics of AIDS
by Philip M. Kayal
1993; 275 pages; Westview Press
ISBN: 0-8133-1729-0

AIDS: Cultural Analysis—Cultural Activism
edited by Douglas Crimp
1988; 275 pages; $13.95; M I T Press
ISBN: 0-262-53079-1

MISCELLANEOUS

Journal Graphics Health and Well-Being Index
(Provides inexpensive transcripts of most TV programs, particularly news and information shows)
Contact Journal Graphics at (303) 831-6400 with program name, air date, topic.

Dictionary of AIDS-Related Terminology
edited by Jeffrey T. Huber
1992; 175 pages; $39.95; Neal-Schuman
ISBN: 1-55570-117-5

Legal Guide for Lesbian and Gay Couples, Seventh Revised Edition
by Hayden Curry and Denis Clifford
1992; 360 pages; $21.95; Nolo Press
ISBN: 0-87337-199-2

Dancing on the Moon: Short Stories about AIDS
by Jameson Currier
1993; 188 pages; $20.00; Viking/Penguin
ISBN: 0-670-84656-2

Purple Heart
by Michael Callen
Available for $15.00 for CD or $10.00 cassette (plus $2.00 shipping and handling per item) from Significant Others Records, Post Office Box 1341, Old Chelsea Station, New York, NY 10113.

NATIONAL AND REGIONAL RESOURCES

ABBREVIATIONS OF SERVICES PROVIDED

Med	Medical Services
Support	Psychological/Spiritual/Religious/ Emotional/Support
Housing	Residential Care/Hospice/Subsidized Housing
Food	Food/Hot Lunch/Meals-on-Wheels
Care	Home Care Buddies
Info	Information/Education
Publish	Published Books/Pamphlets/Newsletters
Policy	Political/Lobbyist/Policy
Legal	Legal Services
$	Financial/Insurance/Viatical
Pharm	Pharmacy/Drug Buyers Club
Sales	Other Sales of HIV-related goods
Other	Other HIV/AIDS Resources
Non-HIV	Other Non-HIV/AIDS-Related Resources

MAGAZINES

AIDS Reports
Post Office Box 14252
Washington, DC 20004

AIDS Treatment News
Hotline: (800) 873-2812

AmFAR Treatment Directory
Hotline: (212) 682-7440

Art and Understanding
Hotline: (800) 841-8707

Being Alive/APLA
Hotline: (213) 667-3262

Beta/San Francisco AIDS Foundation
Hotline: (415) 863-2437

Body Positive
Hotline: (212) 721-1346

Community Prescription Service Infopack
Hotline: (800) 842-0502

Critical Path AIDS Project
Hotline: (215) 545-2212

Diseased Pariah News
Hotline: (510) 891-0455

GMHC Treatment Issues
Hotline: (212) 337-3695

Journal of the Physicians Association for
    AIDS Care
Hotline: (312) 222-1326

Lifetimes II/Stadtlander's Pharmacy
Hotline: (800) 238-7828

Men's Fitness
Office: (818) 884-6800
Fax: (818) 704-5734
21100 Erwin Street
Woodland Hills, CA 91367

Men's Health
Rodale Press
33 E. Minor Street
Emmaus, PA 18098

Notes from the Underground
Hotline: (212) 255-0520

Out Magazine
110 Greene Street, Suite 600
New York, NY 10012

Positive Living/AIDS Project Los Angeles

Hotline: (213) 993-1470

Positively Aware/TPA Network
Hotline: (312) 404-8726

POZ Magazine
Office: (212) 242-2163
Post Office Box 1279
Old Chelsea Station
New York, NY 10113-1279

Praxis
Hotline: (213) 660-7563

Project Inform Perspectives
Hotline: (800) 822-7422

PWA Newsline
Hotline: (800) 828-3280

Step Perspectives
Hotline: (800) 869-7837

The Advocate
Office: (800) 827-0561
Post Office Box 4371
Los Angeles, CA 90078

Women Being Alive
Hotline: (213) 667-2735

OTHER BOOK LISTS

*The following organizations will be happy to
send you their latest HIV/AIDS reading list.
Please send a stamped, self-addressed enve-
lope along with a short note requesting this
list.*

Lambda Rising
Office: (202) 462-6969
1625 Connecticut Avenue NW
Washington, DC 20009-1013

Living Positively
Office: (800) 872-4448
Fax: (212) 929-0822
175 Fifth Avenue
2359
New York, NY 10010

Exceptional Cancer Patients
Office: (203) 343-5950
Fax: (203) 343-5956
300 Plaza Middlesex
Middletown, CT 06457
Services Provided: Support

PHARMACIES AND DRUG BUYERS' CLUBS

American Preferred Plan (APP)
Hotline: (800) 277-9687
Office: (516) 845-5300
Fax: (516) 845-5310
Post Office Box 9019
Farmingdale, NY 11735-9019
Services Provided: Pharm, Sales

Community Prescription Service
Hotline: (800) 842-0502
Office: (212) 229-9102
Fax: (212) 229-9108
349 W. 12th Street, 2nd Floor
New York, NY 10014
Services Provided: Info, Pharm

Healing Alternatives Foundation
Office: (415) 626-4053
Fax: (415) 626-0451
1748 Market Street
San Francisco, CA 94102
Services Provided: Pharm

Priority Pharmacy
Hotline: (800) 487-7115
Fax: (800) 487-7118

3935 First Avenue
San Diego, CA 92103
Services Provided: Info, Publish, Pharm

PWA Health Group (Buyers Club)
Hotline: (212) 255-0520
Office: (212) 255-0520
Fax: (212) 255-2080
150 W. 26th Street
#201
New York, NY 10001
Services Provided: Publish, Policy, Pharm

PX Drugstore
Hotline: (800) 752-5721
5160 Vineland Avenue
North Hollywood, CA 91601
Services Provided: Pharm

Stadtlanders Pharmacy
Hotline: (800) 238-7828
Fax: (412) 825-0589
600 Penn Center Boulevard
Pittsburgh, PA 15235
Services Provided: Info, Publish, Pharm

Sutcliffe Pharmacy
Office: (312) 525-0081
801 W. Irving Park Road
Chicago, IL 60613
Services Provided: Med, Care, Info, $, Pharm

The Medicine Shoppe
Hotline: (800) 578-7294
86 Route 303
Tappan, NY 10983

VIATICAL/ACCELERATED BENEFITS

Ability Life Trust
Hotline: (800) 632-0555
Office: (407) 629-0500
Fax: (407) 629-0599
1177 Louisiana Avenue
Suite 212
Winter Park, FL 32789

Accelerated Benefits Capital
Hotline: (800) 327-8222
Office: (810) 559-9112
Fax: (800) 327-8222
15919 W. Ten Mile Road
#213
Southfield, MI 48075

Accelerated Benefits of Washington, DC
Hotline: (800) 227-8447
Office: (703) 406-2444
Fax: (703) 408-2496
37 Pidgeon Hill Drive
Suite 120
Sterling, VA 20165

American Life Resources
(call collect)
LA Office: (310) 657-8595
SF Office: (415) 986-2432
Fax: (415) 989-1204
50 California Street
#3300
San Francisco, CA 94111

Benefit Advocates
Hotline: (800) 435-8891
Office: (415) 380-8880

180 Montgomery Street
Suite 2180
San Francisco, CA 94104

Benefit Advocates
Hotline: (800) 435-8891
Office: (805) 541-8899
Fax: (805) 641-9001
599 Higuera Street
Suite H
San Luis Obispo, CA 93401
Services Provided: $

Benefits for Life (East Coast)
Hotline: (800) 838-3263
Office: (212) 695-3121
Fax: (212) 695-3203
141 W. 28th Street
#1102
New York, NY 10001

Benefits for Life (West Coast)
Hotline: (800) 838-2363
Office: (415) 331-2363
Fax: (415) 331-2377
475 Gate Five Road
Suite 216
Sausalito, CA 94965
Services Provided: $

Dedicated Resources
Hotline: (800) 677-5026

Dignity Partners
Office: (702) 831-4777
Post Office Box 8819
Incline Village, NV 89452

Estate Trust Co., Inc.
Hotline: (800) 456-5100
Office: (410) 828-1171

Fax: (410) 296-2114
7400 York Road
#300
Baltimore, MD 21204

FT Viatical Settlement Partners
Office: (415) 421-3089
Fax: (415) 421-2133
One Maritime Plaza
#1250
San Francisco, CA 94111

Individual Benefits, Inc.
Office: (910) 299-5100
Fax: (910) 299-9932
624 Guilford College Road
Suite "L"
Greensboro, NC 27409

Kelco, Inc.
Office: (606) 223-3262
Fax: (606) 255-1112
1018 New Circle Road
#204
Lexington, KY 40506

Legacy Benefits Corporation
Hotline: (800) 875-1000
Office: (212) 643-1190
Fax: (212) 643-1180
225 W. 34th Street
#1500
New York, NY 10122

Life Entitlements Corporation
Office: (800) 420-1420
Fax: (212) 775-8039
Four World Trade Center
#5270
New York, NY 10048

Life Funding Corporation
Hotline: (800) 456-8789
Office: (404) 518-8830

Fax: (404) 518-8863
8300 Dunwoody Place
#220
Atlanta, GA 30360

Life Today, Inc.
Hotline: (800) 467-2518
Office: (713) 977-5433
Fax: (713) 977-5817
2401 Fountainview
#900
Houston, TX 77067

Lifetime Options, Inc.
Hotline: (800) 999-5419
Office: (703) 379-8906
Fax: (703) 931-2034
2 Wisconsin Circle
#700
Chevy Chase, MD 20815

Medical Escrow Society
Hotline: (800) 422-1314
Fax: (904) 343-3004
206 North Texas Avenue
#3
Tavares, FL 32778

National Capital Benefits Corporation
Office: (212) 750-1000
Fax: (212) 750-8860
540 Madison Avenue
#1702
New York, NY 10022

National Viatical Association
Hotline: (800) 741-9465
Fax: (817) 741-9466
6614 Sanger
#3
Waco, TX 76710

National Viator Representatives, Inc.
Hotline: (800) 932-0050
Office: (212) 586-5600
Fax: (212) 246-2319
56 W. 57 Street
4th Floor
New York, NY 10019

Neuma (Corporate Office)
Hotline: (800) 457-7828
1007 Church Street
Suite 314
Evanston, IL 60201-5912

Neuma (Dallas Office)
Hotline: (800) 817-3741
Office: (214) 528-9988
3102 Oak Lawn Drive
#700
Dallas, TX 75219

Page & Associates, Inc.
Hotline: (800) 572-4346
5311 Northfield Road
#200
Bedford Heights, OH 44146

The Access Program
Office: (310) 557-1702
Fax: (310) 556-7782
10100 Santa Monica Boulevard
Suite 420
Los Angeles, CA 90067

Viatical Assistance Corporation
Hotline: (800) 892-1282
Office: (817) 772-3888
Fax: (817) 772-6628
Post Office Box 23434
Waco, TX 76702-3434

Viatical Clearing House, Inc.
Hotline: (800) 969-0509

Office: (513) 583-0060
Fax: (513) 583-1478
852 Oak Canyon Drive
Loveland, OH 45140

Viatical Settlements Funding, Inc.
Office: (916) 583-0200
Fax: (916) 583-3618
Post Office Box 3000
Olympic Valley, CA 96148

Viatical Settlements, Inc.
Hotline: (800) 785-7183
Office: (816) 483-6625
Fax: (816) 483-9211
6455 E. Commerce
#170
Kansas City, MO 64120

NATIONAL RESOURCES

ACLU AIDS Project
Office: (212) 944-9800
Fax: (212) 869-9061
132 W. 43rd Street
New York, NY 10036
Services Provided: Legal

ACLU's Lesbian and Gay Rights Project
Hotline: (212) 944-9800
132 W. 43rd Street
New York, NY 10036

AIDS Action Council
Hotline: (202) 986-1300
1875 Connecticut Avenue NW
#700
Washington, DC 20009

AIDS Action Council
2033 M Street NW
#802,
Washington, DC 20036

AIDS Clinical Trials Information Service
Hotline: (800) TRIALS-A (874-2572)
Office: (800) 243-7012
TTY/TDD Fax: (301) 738-6616
Post Office Box 6421
Rockville, MD 20849-6421
Services Provided: Info, Other

AIDS in Prison Project
Office: (202) 234-4830
Fax: (202) 234-4890
1875 Connecticut Avenue NW
Washington, DC 20009
*Services Provided: Info, Publish, Policy,
Legal, Sales, Other*

AIDS Information Network
Office: (215) 922-5120
Fax: (215) 922-6762
32 N. 3rd Street
Philadelphia, PA 19106
Services Provided: Info, Publish

AIDS Project Los Angeles (APLA)
Hotline: (800) 922-2437
1313 N. Vine Street
Los Angeles, CA 90028

AIDS Treatment and Data Network
Hotline: (212) 268-4196
259 W. 30th Street, 9th Floor
New York, NY 10001

AIDS Treatment News
Hotline: (800) 873-2812
Office: (415) 255-0717
Fax: (415) 255-4659
Post Office Box 411256
San Francisco, CA 94141
Services Provided: Publish

American Federation of Home Health
  Agencies
1320 Fenwick Lane
Suite 500
Silver Spring, MD 20910

American Medical Association
515 State Street
Chicago, IL 60610

American Psychological Association
  Office on AIDS
1200 17th Street NW
Washington, DC 20036

American Public Health Association
Office: (202) 789-5688
1015 15th Street NW
Washington, DC 20005
Services Provided: Publish, Policy, Non-HIV

American AIDS PAC
Office: (202) 462-8061
1775 T Street
Washington, DC 20009

American Association for Continuing
  Care
1101 Connecticut Avenue NW
Washington, DC 20036

American Dietetic Organization
Office: (312) 899-0040
216 W. Jackson Boulevard
Chicago, IL 60606-6995

American Red Cross
Office: (202) 973-6000
Fax: (202) 973-6043
Office of HIV/AIDS Education
431 18th Street NW
Washington, DC 20006
Services Provided: Info

AmFAR—American Foundation for AIDS
 Research
Hotline: (212) 682-7440
733 Third Avenue, 12th Floor
New York, NY 10017

CDC, AIDS Activity Office
1600 Clifton Road, Building 3
Room 5B-1
Atlanta, GA 30307-0528

CDC National AIDS/HIV Hotline
Hotline: (800) 342-AIDS
(342-2437)
Office: (800) 344-SIDA (Spanish)

CDC National Sexually Transmitted
 Diseases Hotline
Hotline: (800) 227-8922
Centers for Disease Control
Hotline: (404) 639-2891
Atlanta, GA 30333

CFID Association of America
Hotline: (800) 442-3437
Office: (704) 364-0016
Fax: (704) 365-9755
Post Office Box 220398
Charlotte, NC 28222
Services Provided: Info, Publish

HospiceLink
Hotline: (800) 331-1620
Office: (203) 767-1620
Fax: (203) 767-2746
190 Westbrook Road
Essex, CT 06426
Services Provided: Support, Info, Publish,
Other, Non-HIV

Interfaith Conference/Metropolitan
Washington Task Force on AIDS
1419 V Street NW
Washington, DC 20009

Lambda Legal Defense and Education
 Fund
Hotline: (212) 995-8585
666 Broadway, 12th Floor
New York, NY 10012

NAMES Project
2362 Market Street
San Francisco, CA 94114

National Association Protection and
 Advocacy System
900 2nd Street NE
Suite 211
Washington, DC 20002

National Coalition Hispanic Health and
 Human Services
1030 15th Street NW
Suite 1053
Washington, DC 20005

National Council on Alcoholism and
 Drug Dependency
Hotline: (800) NCA-CALL
Fax: (212) 545-1690
12 W. 21st Street
New York, NY 10001
Services Provided: Info, Publish, Non-HIV

National Gay and Lesbian Task Force
1734 14th Street NW
Washington, DC 20009

National Latina/o Lesbian and Gay
 Organization
Office: (202) 544-0092
Fax: (202) 544-2228
703 G Street SE
Washington, DC 20003
Services Provided: Info, Publish, Policy

National Lawyers Guild AIDS Network
558 Capp Street
San Francisco, CA 94110

National Migrant Resource Program
1515 S. Capitol of Texas Highway
Suite 220
Austin, TX 78746-6544
Services Provided: Info, Publish

National Native American AIDS
   Prevention Center
Office: (510) 444-2051
3515 Grand Avenue
Suite 100
Oakland, CA 94610
Services Provided: Info

National Organization of Black County
   Officials AIDS Education Project
Building C
1631 E. 120th Street
Los Angeles, CA 90059

National Parents Resource Institute
50 Hurt Plaza
Hurt Building
Suite 210
Atlanta, GA 30303

National Task Force on AIDS
   Prevention
273 Church Street
San Francisco, CA 94114

National Academy of Sciences
   Committee/National Strategy for AIDS
2101 Constitution Avenue NW
Washington, DC 20418

National AIDS Bereavement Center
4300 N. Old Dominion Drive
Suite 803
Arlington, VA 22207-3246

National AIDS Hotline for the Hearing
   Impaired
Hotline: (800) 243-7889 (TDD)

National Association for Home Care
519 C Street NE
Washington, DC 20036

National Association of People with AIDS
Hotline: (202) 898-0414
Office: (202) 898-0414
Fax: (202) 898-0435
1413 K Street NW, 8th Floor
Washington, DC 20005
Services Provided: Info, Publish, Policy,
Other

National Association of PWAs
Office: (202) 898-0414
1413 K Street NW
Washington, DC 20005

National Association of Social Workers
Lesbian and Gay Issues
Office: (202) 408-8600
750 First Street NE
Washington, DC 20002

National Education Association
Office: (202) 822-7570
Fax: (202) 822-7775
1201 16th Street NW
Washington, DC 20036
Services Provided: Info, Publish, Non-HIV

National Hospice Organization
Hotline: (800) 658-8898
Office: (703) 243-5900
Fax: (703) 525-5762
1901 N. Moore Street
Suite 901
Arlington, VA 22209
Services Provided: Info, Publish, Policy,
Other, Non-HIV

National Leadership Coalition on AIDS
Office: (202) 429-0930
Fax: (202) 872-1977
1730 M Street NW
Suite 905
Washington, DC 20036

National Lesbian and Gay Health
   Federation
Post Office Box 65472
Washington, DC 20035

National Lesbian and Gay Health
   Foundation
Hotline: (202) 797-3578
1407 S Street NW
Washington, DC 20009

National Minority AIDS Council
Office: (202) 544-1076
300 I Street NE
#400
Washington, DC 20002

National Native American AIDS Hotline
Hotline: (800) 283-2437

National Victim Center
Hotline: (800) FYI-CALL
Office: (817) 877-3355
Fax: (817) 877-3396
307 W. 7th Street
Suite 1001
Fort Worth, TX 76102
Services Provided: Info, Publish

NIH—National Institutes of Health
   Clinical Trials Division
Hotline: (800) 874-2572
Office: (301) 496-4891
Post Office Box 6421
Rockville, MD 20849-6421

Nutritional Health Alliance
Hotline: (800) 226-4NHA
Office: (703) 359-0454
Fax: (703) 359-9343
Box 25317
Washington, DC 20007-8317

Physicians Association for AIDS Care
Office: (312) 222-1326
Fax: (312) 222-0329
101 W. Grand Avenue
#200
Chicago, IL 60610.
Services Provided: Publish

Planned Parenthood Federation of
   America
810 Seventh Avenue
New York, NY 10019

Project Inform (Treatment Information)
Hotline: (800) 822-7422
Office: (415) 558-8669
Fax: (415) 558-0684
1965 Market Street
#220
San Francisco, CA 94103
Services Provided: Publish, Policy

PWA Coalition
Hotline: (212) 647-1415
Office: (800) 828-3280
50 W. 17th Street, 8th Floor
New York, NY 10011

SIECUS
Office: (212) 819-9770
Fax: (212) 819-9776
130 W. 42nd Street
Suite 2500
New York, NY 10036
*Services Provided: Info, Publish, Policy,
Other*

U.S. Centers for Disease Control
    Division of Epidemiology
Hotline: (919) 733-7301
Post Office Box 27687
Raleigh, NC 27611-7687

WHO Collaborating Centre on AIDS
c/o Centers for Disease Control
1600 Clifton Road NE
Atlanta, GA 30333

LOCAL AIDS SERVICES ORGANIZATIONS

Alabama

AIDS Task Force of Alabama
Hotline: (205) 591-4448
Office: (205) 592-2437
Fax: (205) 592-4998
Post Office Box 55703
Birmingham, AL 35255
Services Provided: Housing, Info, Publish, Policy

Cullman County AIDS Task Force
Post Office Box 1678
Cullman, AL 35055

Mobile AIDS Support Services
120B N. Lafayette
Mobile, AL 36604

Montgomery AIDS Outreach
Hotline: (205) 269-1002
Office: (205) 269-1432
Post Office Box 5213
Montgomery, AL 36103
Services Provided: Med, Support, Food, Care, Info, Publish, Other

Alaska

AIDS Program/Anchorage
3601 C Street
Suite 576
Anchorage, AK 99524

Alaskan AIDS Assistance Association
Hotline: (907) 276-4880
1057 Firewood
Anchorage, AK 99503
Services Provided: Support, Housing, Food, Care, Info, Publish, Policy, Legal, Other, Non-HIV

Arizona

Arizona AIDS Info. Line
Hotline: (602) 234-2752
Office: (602) 234-2752
Post Office Box 16423
Phoenix, AZ 85011
Services Provided: Info, Other

Arizona AIDS Project
Office: (602) 265-3300
Fax: (602) 265-9951
4460 N. Central Avenue
Phoenix, AZ 85012
Services Provided: Support, Food, Care, Info, Legal, Other, Non-HIV

PWA Coalition of Tucson
Office: (602) 770-1710
Fax: (602) 622-5822
801 W. Congress
Tucson, AZ 85745
Services Provided: Med, Support, Housing, Food, Info, Publish, Policy, Legal, Pharm, Other

Tucson AIDS Project
Hotline: (602) 322-6226
151 S. Tucson Boulevard
#252
Tucson, AZ 85716

Arkansas

AIDS Support Group
210 Pulaski
Little Rock, AR 72201

Arkansas AIDS Project
Hotline: (501) 663-7833
Fax: (501) 664-5403
5911 H Street
Little Rock, AR 72205
Services Provided: Info, Med, Other

Washington County AIDS Task Force
Hotline: (501) 443-AIDS
Office: (501) 443-AIDS
Post Office Box 4224
Fayetteville, AR 72702
Services Provided: Housing, Care, Info, Other

California (Northern)

AIDS Emergency Fund
Hotline: (415) 558-6999
Fax: (415) 558-6990
1540 Market Street
#320
San Francisco, CA 94102-6035
Services Provided: $

AIDS Health Project
Office: (415) 476-6430
Fax: (415) 476-7996
Box 0884
1855 Folsom Street
Suite 506
San Francisco, CA 94143-0884
Services Provided: Support, Info, Publish, Med, Other

AIDS Minority Health Initiative
Office: (510) 763-1872
Fax: (510) 763-3132

1440 Broadway
Suite 209
Oakland, CA 94612
Services Provided: Med, Support, Housing, Care, Other

AIDS Project/East Bay
Office: (510) 834-8181
Fax: (510) 834-0442
1929 Martin Luther King, Jr. Way
Oakland, CA 94612
Services Provided: Support, Care, Info, Publish, Policy, $, Other

American Indian AIDS Institute
333 Valencia Street, Suite 200
San Francisco, CA 94103

Asian AIDS Project
Office: (415) 227-0946
Fax: (415) 227-0945
300 4th Street
Suite 401
San Francisco, CA 94107
Services Provided: Info, Publish, Sales

Bayview-Hunter's Point Foundation AIDS
    Education Unit
Office: (415) 822-8200
5815 3rd Street
San Francisco, CA 94124

Black Coalition on AIDS
Office: (415) 346-2364
1042 Divisadero Street
San Francisco, CA 94115

Clinic for AIDS and Related Disorders
UCLA Davis Medical Center
2035 Stockton Boulevard
Sacramento, CA 94817

DAIR
2336 Market Street, No. 33
San Francisco, CA 94114

Deaf AIDS Center
Office: (415) 346-8327
Fax: (415) 476-7113
3333 California Street
San Francisco, CA 94118
Services Provided: Support, Info, Other

Division AIDS Activities, S.F.
995 Potrero Avenue
Ward 84
San Francisco, CA 94110

East Bay AIDS Center
Office: (510) 204-1870
Fax: (510) 204-1870
3031 Telegraph Avenue
Berkeley, CA 94705
Services Provided: Support, Med, Other

Face-to-Face
Sonoma County AIDS Network
Office: (707) 887-1581
Fax: (707) 869-1461
Post Office Box 1599
Guerneville, CA 95446
*Services Provided: Support, Care, Info,
Legal, Other*

Gay Men's Health Collective/HIV
2339 Durant Avenue
Berkeley, CA 94704

Haight-Ashbury Free Clinics
Office: (415) 565-1905
3330 Geary Boulevard
San Francisco, CA 94118
Services Provided: Support, Info, Med

Impact AIDS Inc.
Office: (415) 861-3397
Fax: (415) 621-3951

3692 18th Street
San Francisco, CA 94110
Services Provided: Publish, Sales

Mobilization against AIDS
Office: (415) 863-4676
Fax: (415) 863-4740
584 Castro Street # B
San Francisco, CA 94114-1465
Services Provided: Info, Policy

Planetree Health Resource Center of San
   Francisco
2040 Webster Street
San Francisco, CA 94115

Planetree Health Resource Center of San
   Jose
98 N. 17th Street
San Jose, CA 95112

Project AWARE
995 Potrero Avenue
Building 90, Ward 95
Room 513
San Francisco, CA 94110

R and E Research Associates
AIDS International/Info Distribution
Post Office Box 2008
Saratoga, CA 95070

Sacramento AIDS Foundation
1900 K Street
Suite 203
Sacramento, CA 95814

Sacramento County Health Department
Office: (916) 366-2922
Fax: (916) 366-2388
AIDS Unit, 3701 Branch Center Road
Sacramento, CA 95827
Services Provided: Med, Info, Other

San Francisco AIDS Foundation
25 Van Ness Street
Suite 660
San Francisco, CA 94101-6182

San Joaquin AIDS Foundation
4410 N. Pershing Avenue
Suite C-5
Stockton, CA 95207

San Luis Obispo County AIDS Program
  Education and Prevention Project
Office: (805) 781-4200
12191 Johnson Avenue
San Luis Obispo, CA 93401
Services Provided: Med, Info, Other

Santa Clara County Health Department
  AIDS Program
2220 Moorpark
San Jose, CA 95128

Santa Cruz AIDS Project
Office: (408) 427-3900
Fax: (408) 427-0398
Post Office Box 557
Santa Cruz, CA 95061-0557
*Services Provided: Support, Housing, Food,
Care, Info, Legal, Other*

Shanti Project
Office: (415) 864-2273
Fax: (415) 864-6584
1546 Market Street
San Francisco, CA 94102-6007
Services Provided: Support, Care, Other

Solano County Health Department AIDS
  Program
355 Tuolumne Street
Vallejo, CA 94590

Stanislaus Community AIDS Project
1620 N. Carpenter Road
Suite D43
Modesto, CA 95351

Stop AIDS Project/Sacramento
1931 L Street
Sacramento, CA 95814

Stop AIDS Project/San Francisco
347 Dolores Street
Suite 118
San Francisco, CA 94110

Women's AIDS Network
333 Valencia Street, 4th Floor
San Francisco, CA 94102

California (Southern)

Aid for AIDS
8235 Santa Monica Boulevard
Suite 200
West Hollywood, CA 90046

AIDS:CAP (GLRC)
417 Barbara Street
Suite A18
Santa Barbara, CA 93101

AIDS Healthcare Foundation
1800 N. Argyle, 3rd Floor
Los Angeles, CA 90028

AIDS Project Los Angeles
Hotline: (800) 922-AIDS
Office: (213) 993-1600
Fax: (213) 993-1595
1313 N. Vine Street
Los Angeles, CA 90028
*Services Provided: Support, Care, Info,
Publish, Policy, Legal, $, Other*

AIDS Response Program
Office: (714) 534-0961
Fax: (714) 534-5491
12832 Garden Grove Boulevard
Suite E
Garden Grove, CA 92643
Services Provided: Support, Info, Publish

AIDS Santa Clarita Foundation
Post Office Box 220908
Newhall, CA 91322

AIDS Service Center (ASC)
Hotline: (800) 542-8272
Office: (818) 796-5633
Fax: (818) 796-8198
126 W. Del Mar Boulevard
Pasadena, CA 91105
Services Provided: Support, Care, Info, Legal

AIDS Services
County Health Care Services
300 N. San Antonio Road
Santa Barbara, CA 93110

AIDS Services Foundation
17982 Sky Park Circle
Suite J
Irvine, CA 92714-1010

Asian Pacific AIDS Intervention Team
Office: (213) 353-6035
Fax: (213) 413-1539
1313 W. 8th Street
Suite 224
Los Angeles, CA 90017
Services Provided: Support, Info

Being Alive/Long Beach
Hotline: (310) 434-9022
Office: (310) 434-9022
994 Redondo Avenue
Long Beach, CA 90804-5191
Services Provided: Info, Publish

Being Alive/San Diego
Hotline: (619) 291-1400
3960 Park Boulevard
Suite E
San Diego, CA 92103-3506

Black G and L Leadership Forum/AIDS
  Prevention
Hotline: (800) TREAT-HIV
Office: (213) 964-7820
Fax: (213) 964-7830
1219 S. La Brea Avenue
Los Angeles, CA 90019
Services Provided: Support, Info

Caring for Babies with AIDS
Post Office Box 351535
Los Angeles, CA 90035
Services Provided: Support, Housing, Care

Central Valley AIDS Team
Hotline: (209) 264-AIDS
Fax: (209) 265-4716
Post Office Box 4640
Fresno, CA 93744
*Services Provided: Support, Housing, Care,
Info, Publish, Policy, Legal, $, Other, Non-
HIV*

Computerized AIDS Information Network
1213 N. Highland Avenue
Hollywood, CA 90038

Desert AIDS Project
Office: (619) 323-2118
750 S. Vella Road
Palm Springs, CA 92264
*Services Provided: Med, Support, Care, Info,
Publish, Legal, Other*

El Centro Human Services Organization
  Milagros AIDS Project
741 S. Atlantic Boulevard
Los Angeles, CA 90022

Foothill AIDS Project
Hotline: (800) HIV-8058
Office: (909) 920-9265
Fax: (909) 920-4139
8880 Benson Avenue

Suite 114
Montclair, CA 91763
Services Provided: Support, Publish, Care,
Housing, Legal, Food, Info, $, Pharm,
Other

Hollywood Supports
8455 Beverly Boulevard
Suite 305
Los Angeles, CA 90048

Inland AIDS Project
Office: (909) 784-2437
1240 Palmyrita Avenue #E
Riverside, CA 92507

L.A. Shanti
Office: (213) 962-8197
Fax: (213) 962-8299
1616 N. La Brea Avenue
Los Angeles, CA 90028
Services Provided: Support

Latino AIDS Project
Office: (213) 660-9680
Fax: (213) 660-6279
1169 N. Vermont Avenue
Los Angeles, CA 90029
Services Provided: Support, Care, Info,
Policy, Legal, $, Other

Los Angeles County Department of
    Health
AIDS Program, 6th Floor
600 S. Commonwealth Avenue
Los Angeles, CA 90005

Louise L. Hay AIDS Support Group
Hay House
Post Office Box 2212
Santa Monica, CA 90406

Minority AIDS Project
Office: (213) 936-4949
5149 W. Jefferson Boulevard
Los Angeles, CA 90016

Pediatric AIDS Foundation
1311 Colorado Avenue
Santa Monica, CA 90404

San Bernadino County Medical Society
952 S. Mount Vernon Avenue
Colton, CA 92324

San Diego AIDS Foundation
Hotline: (619) 686-5000
Office: (619) 686-5050
Fax: (619) 682-3876
4080 Centre Street
San Diego, CA 92103
Services Provided: Support, Housing, Food,
Care, Info, Legal, Other

Search Alliance
Office: (213) 930-8820
Fax: (213) 934-3919
7461 Beverly Boulevard
Suite 304
Los Angeles, CA 90036
Services Provided: Other

Shanti Project
Hotline: (714) 494-1446
Fax: (714) 497-0543
312 Broadway
Suite 101
Laguna Beach, CA 92651
Services Provided: Support, Food, Care, Info,
Publish

Women's AIDS Project
8240 Santa Monica Boulevard
Los Angeles, CA 90046

Colorado

Boulder County AIDS Project
Hotline: (303) 444-6121
Fax: (303) 444-0260

2118 14th Street
Boulder, CO 80302
Services Provided: Support, Housing, $,
Food, Care, Info, Legal, Other, Non-HIV

Boulder County AIDS Project
Post Office Box 4375
Boulder, CO 80306

Colorado AIDS Project
Post Office Box 18529
Denver, CO 80218

Colorado AIDS Project (CAP)
Hotline: (303) 830-AIDS
Office: (303) 837-9213
Fax: (303) 837-9213
Post Office Box 18529
Denver, CO 80218
Services Provided: Support, Food, Care, Info,
Legal, $, Other

Denver AIDS Prevention Program
605 Bannock Street
Denver, CO 80204-4507

Southern Colorado AIDS Project
Hotline: (713) 578-9092
Office: (719) 578-9092
Post Office Box 311
Colorado Springs, CO 80901
Services Provided: Med, Support, Care,
Housing, Food, Info, Publish, Other, Non-
HIV

Connecticut

AIDS Project Hartford
Hotline: (203) 247-2437
Office: (203) 523-7699
Fax: (203) 231-1996
30 Arbor Street
Hartford, CT 06106-1209
Services Provided: Support, Care, Info,
Publish, Other

AIDS Project New Haven
Hotline: (203) 624-2437
Office: (203) 624-0947
850 Grand Avenue
Suite 206
New Haven, CT 06511
Services Provided: Support, Food, Care, Info,
Publish, Policy, Other

AIDS Project/GNB
Hotline: (203) 225-6789
Post Office Box 1214
147 W. Main Street
New Britain, CT 06050-1214
Services Provided: Support, Care, Info,
Other, Non-HIV

AIDS Project/Middlesex County
Hotline: (203) 344-3474
Fax: (203) 344-0136
Middletown Department of Health
Middletown, CT 06457
Services Provided: Med, Support, Other,
Care, Info, Publish, Policy, Sales, Non-HIV

AIDS Project/Norwalk
137 East Avenue
Norwalk, CT 06851

Bread and Roses
Office: (203) 544-9200
Fax: (203) 544-9539
Post Office Box 363
Georgetown, CT 06829
Services Provided: Support, Housing, Info

Bridgeport AIDS Advisory Committee
2710 North Avenue
Bridgeport, CT 06604

Danbury Health Department
   AIDS Program
Hotline: (203) 796-1613
Office: (203) 796-1613

20 West Street
Danbury, CT 06810
Services Provided: Support, Info

Greenwich Department of Health
Office of HIV Information and Services
Hotline: (203) 622-6496
Fax: (203) 622-7770
101 Field Point Road
Greenwich, CT 06836-2540
Services Provided: Support, Care, Info,
Publish, Policy, Legal, $, Other

Hartford Gay and Lesbian Health
    Collective
Post Office Box 2094
520 Albany Avenue
Hartford, CT 06145-2094

Hispanic Unidos Contra
EL SIDA/AIDS
263 Grand Avenue
New Haven, CT 06513

Mid-Fairfield AIDS Project
30 France Street
Norwalk, CT 06851

New London AIDS Educational Services
Health Department
120 Broad Street
New London, CT 06320

Norwalk Health Department
AIDS Program
137 East Avenue
Norwalk, CT 06851

NW Connecticut AIDS Project
Office: (203) 482-1596
100 Migeon Avenue
Torrington, CT 06790

Stamford Health Department/AIDS
    Program
888 Washington Boulevard
8th Floor
Stamford, CT 06904-2152
Services Provided: Support, Info, Other

Waterbury Department of Health AIDS
    Program
402 E. Main Street
Waterbury, CT 06702

Delaware

Delaware Lesbian/Gay Health Advocates
Hotline: (302) 652-6776
601 Delaware Avenue
Wilmington, DE 19801

Florida

AIDS Help
Post Office Box 4374
Key West, FL 33041

AIDS Prevention/ Key West
Office: (305) 292-6701
Fax: (305) 292-6831
517 Whitehead Street
Key West, FL 33040
Services Provided: Other

Bay County Public Health Unit
605 N. MacArthur Avenue
Panama City, FL 32401

Big Bend CARES
Office: (904) 656-AIDS
Fax: (904) 942-6402
Post Office Box 14365
Tallahassee, FL 32317
Services Provided: Med, Support, $,
Housing, Food, Care, Info, Publish

Central Florida AIDS Unified Resources
Post Office Box 3725
Orlando, FL 32802
Services Provided: Support, Housing, Food,
Care, Info, Publish, Other

Cure AIDS Now, Inc.
Office: (305) 375-0400
Fax: (305) 375-8440
111 SW 3rd Street, 2nd Floor
Miami, FL 33130
Services Provided: Support, Food, Info,
Other

Escambia AIDS Services and Education
1200 W. Leonard Street
Room 318
Pensacola, FL 32501

Florida HIV/AIDS Hotline
Hotline: (800) FLA-AIDS
Office: (904) 681-9131
Post Office Box 20169
Tallahassee, FL 32316
Services Provided: Support, Info, Other

Health Council of West Central Florida
9721 Executive Center Drive North
Suite #114
St. Petersburg, FL 33702-2438

Health Crisis Network
Hotline: (305) 751-7751
Office: (305) 751-7775
Fax: (305) 756-7880
5050 Biscayne Boulevard
Miami, FL 33137
Services Provided: Support, Care, Info, Other

Hope and Help Center of Central Florida
Office: (407) 648-4673
Fax: (407) 648-5688
369 N. Orange Avenue
Orlando, FL 32801
Services Provided: Support, Care, Info,
Publish, Legal, $, Med, Other

HRS/Hillsborough County Health
Department AIDS Program
1112B Kennedy Boulevard
Tampa, FL 33675-5135

Lee County AIDS Task Force
2231 McGregor Boulevard
Fort Myers, FL 33901

Miami AIDS Project (University of
Miami)
Hotline: (305) 547-3838
1800 NW Tenth Avenue, 1st Floor
Miami, FL 33136

North Central Florida AIDS Network
Hotline: (800) 824-6745
Office: (904) 372-4370
Fax: (904) 372-8583
1204 NW. 13 Street
#400
Gainesville, FL 32601
Services Provided: Support, Care, Info,
Publish, Legal, Other

Tampa AIDS Network
Hotline: (813) 978-8683
Office: (813) 979-1919
Fax: (813) 978-3515
11215 N. Nebraska Avenue
#B-3
Tampa, FL 33612
Services Provided: Support, Housing, Care,
Info, Publish, Policy, Other

Georgia

AID-Atlanta
Hotline: (404) 872-0600
1132 W. Peachtree Street NW
Atlanta, GA 30309

AIDS Survival Project
Office: (404) 874-7926
Fax: (404) 872-1192
44 Twelfth Street NE

Atlanta, GA 30309
Services Provided: Info, Publish, Other

Coastal Area Support Team
Post Office Box 2356
Brunswick, GA 31521-2111

Hawaii

Big Island AIDS Project
75-5766 Kuakini Highway
Suite 101
Kailua-Kona, HI 96740

Gay Community Center
1154 Fort Street Mall
Suite 415
Honolulu, HI 96801

Life Foundation
Hotline: (808) 971-2437
Office: (808) 971-2437
Fax: (808) 971-7850
Post Office Box 88980
Honolulu, HI 96830
Services Provided: Support, Legal Policy, Care, Info, Publish, Food, Other, Non-HIV

Malama Pono/Kauai AIDS Project
Post Office Box 1500
Kapaa, HI 96746

Waikiki Health Center
277 Ohua Avenue
Honolulu, HI 96815

Idaho

Idaho AIDS Foundation
Hotline: (208) 345-2277
Post Office Box 421
Boise, ID 83701-4321

Idaho Department of Health and Welfare
Health Division
AIDS Program
450 W. State Street
Boise, ID 83720

Illinois

AIDS Care Network
Office: (815) 968-5181
221 N. Longwood
Suite 105
Rockford, IL 61107-4168
Services Provided: Support, Housing, Food, Care, Info, Publish, Legal, Pharm, Med, Other

AIDS Foundation Chicago
Hotline: (312) 642-5454
1332 N. Halstead
#303
Chicago, IL 60622

Cook County Hospital AIDS Service
1835 W. Harrison Street
Chicago, IL 60612

Gay Community AIDS Project
Hotline: (217) 351-AIDS
Office: (217) 351-AIDS
Post Office Box 713
Champaign, IL 61820
Services Provided: Support, Housing, Care, Info, Publish, Other

Hispanic Health Alliance
Office: (312) 252-6888
Fax: (312) 252-0990
1579 N. Milwaukee
Suite 230
Chicago, IL 60622
Services Provided: Housing, Info, Publish

Horizons Community Services
Hotline: (800) AID-AIDS
Office: (312) 472-6469
Fax: (312) 472-6643
961 W. Montana
Chicago, IL 60614
Services Provided: Support, Info, Legal, Non-HIV

Howard Brown Health Center
Hotline: (312) 871-5777
945 W. George Street
Chicago, IL 60657

Midwest Hispanic AIDS Coalition
Coalicion Hispana Sobre el SIDA del Medioeste
Office: (312) 772-8195
1753 N. Damen
Chicago, IL 60647

Indiana

Damien Center
Office: (317) 632-0123
Fax: (317) 632-4362
1350 N. Pennsylvania
Indianapolis, IN 46202
Services Provided: Support, Housing, Legal, Publish, Food, Care, Info, Other, Non-HIV

Indiana Community AIDS Action Network
Hotline: (317) 920-3190
3951 N. Meridian
Suite 200
Indianapolis, IN 46208

Indiana State Board of Health AIDS Office
Hotline: (800) 848-2437
Fax: (317) 633-0663
1330 W. Michigan Street
Indianapolis, IN 46206

Services Provided: Info, Publish, Policy, Other, Non-HIV

Madison/Delaware County AIDS Task Force
Hotline: (800) 659-9908
Office: (317) 646-9206
Fax: (317) 646-9208
1160 Meridian Plaza
Suite 640
Anderson, IN 46016
Services Provided: Support, Food, Info, Other

Project AIDS Lafayette
Office: (317) 742-2305
Post Office Box 5375
810 North Street
Lafayette, IN 47903
Services Provided: Support, Food, Care, Info, Legal, Other

Iowa

Iowa Center for AIDS Resources and Education
Office: (319) 338-2135
Post Office Box 3989
Iowa City, IA 52244
Services Provided: Support, Care, Info, Publish, $, Other

Iowa Department of Public Health STD/HIV
Hotline: (800) 445-AIDS
Office: (515) 281-4936
Fax: (515) 281-4529
Lucas Building, 1st Floor
Des Moines, IA 50319
Services Provided: Support, Food, Info, Publish, Med, Other, Non-HIV

Johnson County AIDS Project
1105 Gilbert Court
Iowa City, IA 52240

Rapids AIDS Project
Hotline: (319) 393-9579
Office: (319) 393-3500
Fax: (319) 393-1841
c/o American Red Cross
3601 42nd Street NE
Cedar Rapids, IA 52402
Services Provided: Support, Food, Care, Info, Publish

Kansas

Topeka AIDS Project
Office: (913) 232-3100
Fax: (913) 232-3186
1915 SW 6th Street
Topeka, KS 66604-4726
Services Provided: Support, Care, Info, Other

Kentucky

AIDS Education Coalition, Inc.
850 Barret Avenue
Suite 301
Louisville, KY 40204

AIDS Southern Kentucky
Office: (615) 842-5833
Post Office Box 9733
Bowling Green, KY 42102-9733
Services Provided: Support, Housing, Care, Info, Legal, $

AIDS Volunteer
Hotline: (606) 231-7545
Office: (606) 254-2865
Post Office Box 431
Lexington, KY 40585
Services Provided: Support, Housing, $, Care, Info, Publish, Policy, Legal, Other

AIDS/HIV Prevention Program
Room 323, 400 E. Gray Street
Louisville, KY 40202

Lexington-Fayette County Health
   Department
Office: (606) 288-2374
650 Newtown Pike
Lexington, KY 40508
Services Provided: Med, Support, Housing, Info, $, Other

Louisville and Jefferson County Health
   Department AIDS/HIV Prevention
   Program
Post Office Box 1704
Louisville, KY 40201

North Kentucky AIDS Task Force
Office: (502) 341-0696
610 Medical Village Drive
Edgewood, KY 41017
Services Provided: Med, Info, Publish

Louisiana

Central LA AIDS Support Services
Office: (318) 442-1010
824 Sixteenth Street
Alexandria, LA 71301
Services Provided: Support, Food, Care, Info, Publish, Other

Immunological Support Program
Office: (504) 765-8917
5000 Hennessy Boulevard
Baton Rouge, LA 70809
Services Provided: Support, Housing, Info, Other

New Orleans Health Department
Delgado Clinic, 2nd Floor
320 S. Claiborne Avenue
New Orleans, LA 70112

NO/AIDS Task Force
Hotline: (504) 944-AIDS
Office: (504) 945-4000

Fax: (504) 945-4048
1407 Decatur Street
New Orleans, LA 70116-2120
*Services Provided: Med, Support, Food,
Care, Info, Publish, Policy, $, Other*

Maine

The AIDS Project
Hotline: (207) 775-1267
Office: (207) 774-6877
22 Monument Square, 5th Floor
Portland, ME 04101
*Services Provided: Support, Food, Info,
Policy, Other*

Maryland

Chase-Brexton Clinic
241 W. Chase Street
Baltimore, MD 21201

Dorchester County Health Department
Route 1, Box 50, Woods Road
Cambridge, MD 21613

Health Education Resource Organization
Hotline: (410) 945-2437
101 W. Reade Street
Suite 825
Baltimore, MD 21201

Johns Hopkins Hospital First AIDS
   Service
600 N. Wolfe Street
Block 1111
Baltimore, MD 21205

Prince George's County Health
   Department
Office on AIDS
3003 Hospital Drive
Cheverly, MD 20785

Massachusetts

AIDS International Deaf/Tek
Post Office Box 2431
Framingham, MA 0170-0404

AIDS Action Committee
Hotline: (800) 235-2331
Office: (617) 437-6200
131 Clarendon Street
Boston, MA 02116
*Services Provided: Support, Housing, Food,
Care, Info, Publish, Policy, Legal, $, Other*

Clinical AIDS Program
Boston City Hospital
818 Harrison Avenue
Boston, MA 02118

Comprehensive Pediatric AIDS Program
Boston City Hospital
Dowling 5 S
818 Harrison Avenue
Boston, MA 02118

Fenway Community Health Center
16 Haviland Street
Boston, MA 02115

Haitian Coalition on AIDS in
   Massachusetts
177 Harvard Street
Dorchester, MA 02124

La Ahanza Hispana
409 Dudley Street
Roxbury, MA 02119

Massachusetts AIDS Program
150 Tremont Street
Boston, MA 02111

Michigan

Calhoun County AIDS Education Steering
  Committee
190 E. Michigan Avenue
Battle Creek, MI 49107

HIV/AIDS Resource Center
Office: (313) 572-9355
Fax: (313) 572-0554
3075 Clarke Road
#203
Ypsilanti, MI 48197
Services Provided: Support, Care, Info,
Publish, Other

Kalamazoo County AIDS Prevention
  Program
418 W. Kalamazoo Avenue
Kalamazoo, MI 49007

The AIDS Project Detroit Health
  Department
Hotline: (313) 876-0980
1151 Taylor
Detroit, MI 48202

Washtenaw County Public Health, VD
  and AIDS Counseling and Testing
  Clinic
Hotline: (313) 484-6760
Fax: (313) 484-7202
555 Towner Boulevard
Ypsilanti, MI 48198
Services Provided: Med, Support, Info,
Other, Non-HIV

Minnesota

Aliveness Project
Office: (612) 822-7946
Fax: (612) 822-9668
730 E. 38th Street
Minneapolis, MN 55407

Services Provided: Support, Food, Info,
Publish, Other, Non-HIV

Archdiocese/AIDS Ministry Program
Office: (612) 672-4345
Riverside Medical Center
Riverside at 25th Avenue South
Minneapolis, MN 55454

Minnesota AIDS Project
Hotline: (612) 373-AIDS
Office: (612) 341-2060
Fax: (612) 341-4057
1400 Park
Minneapolis, MN 55404
Services Provided: Support, Housing, Care,
Info, Publish, Policy, Legal, Other

Mississippi

Hattiesburg Area AIDS Coalition
Pine Belt Mental Health Center
Post Office Box 1030
Hattiesburg, MS 39403

Mississippi Gay/Lesbian Alliance
Hotline: (601) 371-3019
Post Office Box 8342
Jackson, MS 39284-8342
Services Provided: Med, Support, Care, Info,
Legal, Other, Non-HIV

Mississippi HIV Education and Prevention
Hotline: (601) 960-7723
2423 N. State Street
Box 1700
Jackson, MS 39215-1700

Missouri

AIDS Project of the Ozarks
Office: (417) 881-1900
1722-LL S. Glenstone

Springfield, MO 65804
Services Provided: Med, Support, Care, Info, Publish, $

Four State Community AIDS Project
Post Office Box 3476
Joplin, MO 64803-3476

Good Samaritan AIDS Project
Hotline: (816) 561-8780
3030 Walnut Street
Kansas City, MO 64108

Kansas City Free Health Clinic
Office: (816) 753-5144
Fax: (816) 753-0804
2 E. 39th, 2nd Floor
Kansas City, MO 64111
Services Provided: Med, Support, Info, Publish, Legal, $, Pharm, Non-HIV, Other

Kansas City Regional Hemophilia Center
Office: (816) 235-1820
2301 Holmes
Kansas City, MO 64108
Services Provided: Med, Support, Info

Montana

Yellowstone AIDS Project
Hotline: (406) 245-2029
3308 Second Avenue North
Billings, MT 59101

Nebraska

Douglas County Health Department
1819 Farnam Street
Room 401
Omaha, NE 68183

Nebraska AIDS Project
Hotline: (402) 342-6367

3624 Leavenworth Street
Omaha, NE 68105

Nevada

Aid for AIDS of Nevada
Office: (702) 474-2437
1111 Desert Lane
Las Vegas, NV 89102

Aid for AIDS of Nevada (AFAN)
Hotline: (702) 382-2326
1111 Desert Lane
Las Vegas, NV 89102

Nevada AIDS Foundation
Post Office Box 478
Reno, NV 89504

Nevada State Health Division
Hotline: (702) 687-4800
505 E. King Street
Room 304
Carson City, NV 89710

New Hampshire

New Hampshire AIDS Foundation
Office: (603) 623-0710
Fax: (603) 622-3288
Post Office Box 59
130 Middle Street
Manchester, NH 03105-0059
Services Provided: Support, Housing, Food, Care, Info, Publish, Pharm, Other

New Hampshire Department of Health
Hotline: (603) 271-4502
Health And Welfare Building
6 Hazen Drive
Concord, NH 03301

New Jersey

Hyacinth AIDS Foundation
Hotline: (800) 433-0254
Office: (908) 246-0204
Fax: (908) 246-4137
103 Bayard Street
New Brunswick, NJ 08901
Services Provided: Support, Food, Care, Info, Legal, Other

Hyacinth House (NJ AIDS Organization)
Hotline: (800) 433-0254
700 Park Avenue
Plainfield, NJ 07060

L.I.F.T. AIDS Education/Prevention
  Program for Minorities
225 N. Warren Street
Trenton, NJ 08618

National Pediatric AIDS Resource Center
Hotline: (800) 362-0071
Office: (201) 268-8251
15 S. Ninth Street
Newark, NJ 07107
Services Provided: Info, Publish, Policy

New Mexico

AIDS Prevention Program
1190 St. Francis Drive
Santa Fe, NM 87503

New Mexico AIDS Services
Hotline: (800) 545-2437
Office: (505) 266-0911
Fax: (505) 266-5104
4200 Silver Street SE
Suite D
Albuquerque, NM 87108-2721
Services Provided: Support, Housing, Food, Care, Info, Publish, Policy, Legal

New Mexico AIDS Services
Office: (505) 820-2437
Fax: (505) 820-2100
1229 St. Francis Drive
Suite C
Santa Fe, NM 87505
Services Provided: Support, Housing, Food, Care, Info, Publish, Policy, Legal, $, Other, Non-HIV

New Mexico AIDS Services
124 Quency NE
Albuquerque, NM 87108

Santa Fe Cares
Hotline: (505) 989-9255
Post Office Box 1255
Santa Fe, NM 87504

New York

ACT UP—AIDS Coalition to Unleash
  Power
Hotline: (212) 564-2437
Fax: (212) 989-1797
135 W. 29 Street, 10th Floor
New York, NY 10001

AIDS Center of Queens County
Office: (718) 896-2500
Fax: (718) 275-2094
97-45 Queens Boulevard
Suite 1220
Rego Park, NY 11374
Services Provided: Support, Food, Care, Info, Legal, Other

AIDS Community Services
220 Delaware Avenue
Suite 512
Buffalo, NY 14202-2107

AIDS Comprehensive Family Care Center
Hotline: (718) 430-3333
Office: (718) 430-2940

Fax: (718) 518-7386
Einstein College of Medicine
1300 Morris Park Avenue
Room M-219
Bronx, NY 10461
Services Provided: Med

AIDS Council of N.E. New York
Hotline: (518) 445-AIDS
Office: (518) 434-4686
Fax: (518) 427-8184
88 Fourth Avenue
Albany, NY 12202
Services Provided: Support, Food, Info,
Other

AIDS Education and Resource SUNY
Level 2, Room 075
Health Sciences Center
Stony Brook, NY 11794

AIDS Institute, NY State
Hotline: (212) 613-2432
5 Penn Plaza, Room 407
New York, NY 10001

AIDS Institute, New York State
  Department of Health
Empire State Plaza, Corning Tower
Room 2580
Albany, NY 12237

AIDS Network of West New York, Inc.
Office: (716) 847-0377
121 W. Tupper Street
Buffalo, NY 14201
Services Provided: Info, Other

AIDS Prevention Project for Youth
2340 Amsterdam Avenue
New York, NY 10033

AIDS Project at the Women's Clinic
Hotline: (718) 991-9250

Office: (718) 991-9498
Fax: (718) 991-3829
910 E. 172nd Street
Bronx, NY 10460
Services Provided: Med, Support, Info,
Other, Non-HIV

AIDS Related Community Services
Office: (914) 345-8888
2269 Saw Mill River Road
Building 1 South
Elmsford, NY 10523

AIDS Resource Center
Hotline: (212) 633-2500
275 Seventh Avenue, 12th Floor
New York, NY 10001

AIDS Rochester, Inc.
Hotline: (716) 442-2200
Office: (716) 442-2220
Fax: (716) 442-5049
1350 University Avenue
Rochester, NY 14607
Services Provided: Support, Housing, $,
Food, Care, Info, Publish, Policy, Other

AIDS Theatre Project
Office: (212) 475-6200 x305
c/o The Educational Alliance
197 E. Broadway
U-2
New York, NY 10002
Services Provided: Info, Other

Body Positive
Hotline: (212) 721-1346
Office: (212) 721-1619
Fax: (212) 787-9633
2095 Broadway
New York, NY 10023
Services Provided: Support, Info, Publish,
Other

Brooklyn AIDS Task Force
Hotline: (718) 783-0883
465 Dean Street
Brooklyn, NY 11217

Brooklyn AIDS Task Force Community
    Service Program
22 Chapel Street
Brooklyn, NY 11202

Brooklyn Catholic Charities Office for
    Pastoral Care of the Sick
Office: (718) 722-6112
191 Joralemon Street
Brooklyn, NY 11201
Services Provided: Support

Centerbridge Project
(AIDS Bereavement Group)
Lesbian and Gay Community Services
    Center
Office: (212) 620-7310
Fax: (212) 924-2657
208 W. 13th Street
New York, NY 10011
Services Provided: Support, Info, Publish,
Policy, Other, Non-HIV

Central NY AIDS Task Force
627 W. Genesee Street
Syracuse, NY 13204

Choice in Dying
200 Varick Street
New York, NY 10014-4810

Columbia University
AIDS Prevention and Education Services
600 W. 168th Street
New York, NY 10032

Community Health Project
Office: (212) 675-3559
Fax: (212) 645-0013

208 W. 13th Street
New York, NY 10011
Services Provided: Med, Support, Info,
Other, Non-HIV

Community Research Initiative on AIDS
    (CRIA)
Office: (212) 924-3934
Fax: (212) 924-3936
275 Seventh Avenue
New York, NY 10001
Services Provided: Med, Publish

East End AIDS Wellness Project
Office: (516) 725-5102
55 Main Street
Post Office Box 1357
Sag Harbor, NY 11963
Services Provided: Support, Info

Friends in Deed (Holistic/Non-Medical
    Support)
Hotline: (212) 925-2009
594 Broadway
Suite 706
New York, NY 10012

Gay Men's Health Crisis
Hotline: (212) 807-6655
Office: (212) 645-7470
129 W. 20th Street
New York, NY 10011
Services Provided: Support, Food, Care, Info,
Publish, Policy, Legal

Gaynet
Hotline: (800) 442-9638
Fax: (212) 898-8612
425 E. 61st Street
New York, NY 10021

Health Education AIDS Liaison
Hotline: (800) 410-HEAL
Office: (212) 873-0780

Fax: (212) 873-0891
Post Office Box 1103
Old Chelsea Station
New York, NY 10113
Services Provided: Info, Publish

Health WATCH Information and
    Promotion Service
3020 Glenwood Road
Brooklyn, NY 11210

Hispanic AIDS Forum
121 Avenue of the Americas
5th Floor, Room 505
New York, NY 10013

Housing Works
(for Homeless PWAs/HIV+s)
Hotline: (212) 966-0466
494 Broadway
Suite 700
New York, NY 10012

LIAAC—Long Island Association for
    AIDS Care, Inc.
Hotline: (516) 385-2437
Office: (516) 385-2451
Post Office Box 2859
Huntington Station, NY 11746-0685
*Services Provided: Support, Other, $, Food,
Care, Info, Publish, Policy, Legal*

Minority Task Force on AIDS (Black
    AIDS)
Hotline: (212) 563-8340
505 Eighth Avenue
16th Floor
New York, NY 10018

Monroe County Department of Health
AIDS Coordination Project
111 Westfall Road

Room 946
Rochester, NY 14693

Monroe County Medical Society
1441 East Avenue
Rochester, NY 14610

Nassau County Medical Center AIDS
    Program
2201 Hempstead Turnpike
East Meadow, NY 11554

Northern Lights Alternatives
Office: (212) 765-3202
Fax: (212) 765-2944
601 W. 50th Street
Suite 503
New York, NY 10019
Services Provided: Support

NY City Department of Health,
    AIDS Education
Box 46, 125 Worth Street
New York, NY 10013

NY City Department of Health,
AIDS Programs
Box A/1, 125 Worth Street
New York, NY 10013

Office of Gay and Lesbian Health
    Concerns
125 Worth Street, Box 67
New York, NY 10013

Pediatrics and Pregnancy AIDS Hotline
Hotline: (718) 430-3333
Office: (718) 430-2940
Albert Einstein College of Medicine
1300 Morris Park Avenue
Bronx, NY 10461
Services Provided: Med, Food, Info, Other

People with AIDS Coalition
31 W. 26th Street
New York, NY 10010

Southern Tier AIDS Program
Hotline: (800) 333-0892
Office: (607) 798-1706
Fax: (607) 798-1977
122 Baldwin Street
Johnson City, NY 13790
Services Provided: Support, Info, Publish,
Policy, Other

Staten Island AIDS Task Force
Hotline: (718) 448-2255
Office: (718) 981-3366
25 Hyatt Street, 5th Floor
Staten Island, NY 10301

Treatment Action Group (TAG)
Office: (212) 260-0300
Fax: (212) 260-8561
147 Second Avenue
#601
New York, NY 10003

United Action for AIDS
Office: (212) 337-1227
Fax: (212) 337-1220
175 Fifth Avenue
#2179
New York, NY 10010

Village Nursing Home AIDS Day
Treatment Program
133 W. 20th Street
New York, NY 10011

WARN/Women and AIDS Resource
Network
Hotline: (718) 596-6007
Fax: (718) 596-6041

30 Third Avenue
Brooklyn, NY 11217
Services Provided: Support, Housing, Info,
Policy, Other

West Side AIDS Project
593 Columbus Avenue
New York, NY 10024

Whole Foods Project
Office: (212) 420-1828
Fax: (212) 420-1604
115 E. 23rd Street, 10th Floor
New York, NY 10010
Services Provided: Food

Women and AIDS Research Network
Post Office Box 020525
Brooklyn, NY 11202

North Carolina

AIDS Community Residence Association
   (ACRA)
Hotline: (919) 479-4834
Post Office Box 61584
Durham, NC 27715

AIDS Services Project
Post Office Box 3203
Durham, NC 27705-1203

AIDS Task Force of Winston-Salem
Office: (919) 723-5031
836 Oak Street
Winston-Salem, NC 27101
Services Provided: Support, Food, Care, Info,
Publish, $, Other, Non-HIV

AIDS Task Force of Winston-Salem
Hotline: (919) 723-5031
Post Office Box 20983
Winston-Salem, NC 27120

GROW
(a Community Service Corporation)
Hotline: (919) 675-9222
341-11 S. College Road
#182
Wilmington, NC 28403
Services Provided: Support, Info, Other,
Non-HIV

GROW AIDS Resource Project
Post Office Box 4535
Wilmington, NC 28406

Metrolina AIDS Project (MAP)
Hotline: (704) 333-AIDS
Office: (704) 333-1435
Fax: (704) 376-8794
Post Office Box 32662
Charlotte, NC 28232
Services Provided: Support, Care, Info, Other

Onslow County AIDS Task Force
Hotline: (919) 347-2154
612 College Street
Jacksonville, NC 28540

Stanley County Task Force
945 N. 5th Street
Albemarle, NC 28001

The AIDS Service Agency
Hotline: (919) 834-2437
Fax: (919) 832-8321
Post Office Box 12583
Raleigh, NC 27605
Services Provided: Support, Housing, Food,
Care, Info, Publish, $

The AIDS Services Project (TASP)
Hotline: (919) 286-7475
Post Office Box 3203
Durham, NC 27715-3203

Triad Health Project
Hotline: (919) 275-1654
Post Office Box 5716
Greensboro, NC 27435-071

Western North Carolina AIDS Project
Hotline: (800) 346-3731
Post Office Box 2411
Asheville, NC 28802

North Dakota

North Dakota Department of Health/
  Disease Control
Hotline: (701) 224-2378
600 E. Boulevard Avenue
Bismarck, ND 58505-0200

Ohio

AIDS Advisory Board of Lake County
Hotline: 350-2437
Office: 350-2190
Lake County Health Department
105 Main Street
Painesville, OH 44077
Services Provided: Info, Other

AIDS Volunteers of Cincinnati
Hotline: (513) 421-2437
2183 Central Parkway
Cincinnati, OH 45214
Services Provided: Support, Food, Care, Info,
Publish, Other

Athens AIDS Task Force
Office: (614) 592-4397
18 N. College Street
Athens, OH 45701
Services Provided: Support, Info, Sales,
Other

Auglaize County AIDS Task Force
Auglaize County Health Department

Office: (419) 738-3410
214 S. Wagner Street
Wapakoneta, OH 45895
Services Provided: Info

Cincinnati Health Department
HIV Education and Counseling Site
3101 Burnet Avenue
Cincinnati, OH 45229

Columbus AIDS Task Force
Hotline: (614) 488-2437
1500 W. Third Avenue
Suite 329
Columbus, OH 43212

Dayton Area AIDS Task Force
Post Office Box 3214
Dayton, OH 45401

Erie County General Health District
  AIDS Task Force
420 Superior Street
Erie, OH 44870

Health Issues Task Force
Hotline: (216) 621-0766
2250 Euclid Avenue
Cleveland, OH 44115

Lesbian-Gay Community Service Center
  of Greater Cleveland
Office: (216) 522-1991
Fax: (216) 522-0025
Post Office Box 6177
Cleveland, OH 44101
Services Provided: Support, Info, Publish,
Other, Non-HIV

Mahoning County Area AIDS Task Force
Hotline: (216) 782-2014
Post Office Box 1143
City Hall, 7th Floor
Youngstown, OH 44501

Services Provided: Support, Food, Care, Info,
$, Other

NE Ohio Task Force on AIDS
Post Office Box 44309-2138
251 E. Mill Street
Akron, OH 44309-2138

Southern Ohio AIDS Task Force
Post Office Box 1287
Portsmouth, OH 45662

Stark County AIDS Task Force
Hotline: (216) 489-3423
Office: (216) 489-3231
Fax: (216) 489-3335
420 N. Market
Canton, OH 44702
Services Provided: Other, Non-HIV

Oklahoma

HIV Resource Center
Office: (918) 749-4194
Fax: (918) 749-4213
4154 S. Harvard
Suite H-I
Tulsa, OK 74135
Services Provided: Support, Housing, Info,
Publish, Legal, Other, Non-HIV

Oasis Resources Center
Hotline: (405) 525-2437
2135 NW 39th Street
Oklahoma City, OK 73112

Oklahoma State Department of Health
Hotline: (405) 271-4636
1000 NE Loth Street
Oklahoma City, OK 73117-129

Regional AIDS Interfaith Network
  (RAIN)
Hotline: (918) 749-4195

4151 S. Harvard
Suite H-I
Tulsa, OK 74135

Shanti/Tulsa
Hotline: (918) 749-7898
Post Office Box 4318
Tulsa, OK 74159

Oregon

Cascade AIDS Project
Hotline: (800) 777-2437
Office: (503) 223-5907
620 SW Fifth
#300
Portland, OR 97204
Services Provided: Support, Care, Info,
Publish, Legal, Other

Good Samaritan Hospital
AIDS Task Force
NW 23rd Street
Portland, OR 97120

Multnomah County Health Department
HIV Health Center
Office: (503) 248-5020
Fax: (503) 248-5022
426 SW Stark, 3rd Floor
Portland, OR 97204
Services Provided: Med, Support, Pharm,
Other

Phoenix Rising
Suite 404, 333 SW 5th
Portland, OR 97204

Willamette AIDS Council
329 W. 13th Avenue
Suite D
Eugene, OR 97401

Pennsylvania

Action AIDS
Office: (215) 981-0088
Fax: (215) 854-6735
1216 Arch Street, 4th Floor
Philadelphia, PA 19107
Services Provided: Support, Care, Info,
Publish, Other

AIDS Intervention Project
Post Office Box 352
201 Chestnut Avenue
Altoona, PA 16601

BEBASHI
Office: (215) 457-9050
Fax: (215) 546-6107
1233 Locust
#401
Philadelphia, PA 19107
Services Provided: Med, Support, Care,
Housing, Food, Info, Publish, Policy, Legal

Berks AIDS Network
Hotline: (215) 375-2242
Office: (215) 375-6523
429 Walnut Street
Post Office Box 8626
Reading, PA 19603-8626
Services Provided: Support, Food, Care, Info,
Publish, Policy, Other

CHOICE
Hotline: (215) 545-8686
1642 Pine Street
Philadelphia, PA 19103

Critical Path AIDS Project, Inc.
Hotline: (215) 545-2212
2062 Lombard Street
Philadelphia, PA 19146
Services Provided: Info, Publish, Other

Home Nursing Agency
  AIDS Intravention Project of Central
Pennsylvania
201 Chestnut Avenue
Altoona, PA 16603

PACT
Office: (412) 647-7228
University of Pittsburgh Medical Center
Desoto at O'Hara Street
Pittsburgh, PA 15213
Services Provided: Med

Pennsylvania Department of Health
Hotline: (717) 783-0573
Health and Welfare Building
Room 912
Post Office Box 90
Harrisburg, PA 17108

Persad Center
Office: (412) 441-9786
Fax: (412) 363-2875
5150 Penn Avenue
Pittsburgh, PA 15224-1627
Services Provided: Support, Info

Philadelphia AIDS Hotline
Hotline: (215) 732-2437
1642 Pine Street
Philadelphia, PA 19103

Philadelphia Community Health
  Alternatives
Philadelphia AIDS Task Force
1216 Walnut Street
Philadelphia, PA 19107

Pittsburgh AIDS Task Force
Office: (412) 242-2500
905 West Street, 4th Floor
Pittsburgh, PA 15221-2833
Services Provided: Care, Info, Legal, Other

Pittsburgh Treatment and Evaluation
  Unit
Post Office Box 7526
Pittsburgh, PA 15213
Services Provided: Med

South Central AIDS Assistance
  Network
Office: (717) 238-2437
Fax: (717) 238-1709
2A Kline Village
Suite A
Harrisburg, PA 17104
*Services Provided: Support, Care, Info,
Publish, Legal, Other*

We the People
Office: (215) 545-6868
Fax: (215) 545-8437
425 S. Broad
Philadelphia, PA 19147
*Services Provided: Med, Support, Food,
Housing, Info, Publish, Policy, Pharm,
Other*

YEHSS!
(York Extended Health
  Social Services)
Office: (717) 846-6776
Fax: (717) 854-0377
101 E. Market Street, 2nd Floor
York, PA 17401
*Services Provided: Med, Support, Food,
Care, Info, Policy, Legal, $, Pharm, Other,
Non-HIV*

York Area AIDS Coalition
Office: (717) 846-6776
Fax: (717) 854-0377
c/o YHESS!
101 E. Market Street
York, PA 17401

Puerto Rico

AIDS Central Office/Puerto Rico
  Department
Hotline: (809) 721-2000
Post Office Box 71421
San Juan, PR 00936-8523

Foundacion SIDA de Puerto Rico
Hotline: (809) 782-9600
Fax: (809) 782-1411
G.P.O. Box 36-4842
San Juan, PR 00936-4842
Services Provided: Support, Housing, $,
Care, Info, Publish, Policy, Pharm, Other

Rhode Island

Project AIDS
Hotline: (401) 831-5522
95 Chestnut Street, 3rd Floor
Providence, RI 02908-4161

Stratogen Health
Hotline: (401) 781-2400
Office: (800) 285-8884
Fax: (401) 781-2687
400 Reservoir Avenue
Providence, RI 2907
Services Provided: Med, Support, Care, Info,
Publish, $, Pharm, Other

South Carolina

International Society for AIDS Education
Office: (803) 777-6217
Fax: (803) 777-6217
University of South Carolina,
School of Public Health
Columbia, SC 29208
Services Provided: Info, Publish, Other

Palmetto AIDS Life Support Services
Hotline: (803) 779-7257

Post Office Box 12124
Columbia, SC 29211

South Carolina AIDS Education Network
Hotline: (803) 736-1171
2768 Decker Boulevard
Columbia, SC 29206
Services Provided: Info, Publish, Sales, Non-
HIV

South Carolina Department of Health
  and Environment
HIV/AIDS Division
Hotline: (803) 737-4110
Post Office Box 101106
Columbia, SC 29211

South Dakota

South Dakota Department of Health
  AIDS/HIV
Hotline: (605) 773-3364
445 E. Capital Avenue
Pierre, SD 57501-3185

Tennessee

AIDS Response
Hotline: (615) 523-2437
Post Office Box 6069
Knoxville, TN 37914-6069

AIDS Response Knoxville
Office: (615) 523-2437
Post Office Box 6069
Knoxville, TN 37914

Friends for Life
Hotline: (901) 272-0855
321 S. Bellevue
Memphis, TN 38104

Human Beings Care
Hotline: (800) 562-3383
Office: (901) 423-0330

Post Office Box 3339
Jackson, TN 38303
Services Provided: Support, Care, Info, Other

Nashville Council on AIDS Resources,
    Education and Services
Post Office Box 25107
Nashville, TN 37202

Sullivan County Health Department
Post Office Box 630
Blountville, TN 37617

Tennessee Department of Health
    AIDS Program
Hotline: (615) 741-7500
C20221 Cordell Hull Building
Nashville, TN 37247-4947

Tennessee Hospital Association
Task Force on AIDS
500 Interstate Boulevard South
Nashville, TN 37210

Texas

Abilene AIDS Hotline
Office: (915) 677-2437
401 N. Jefferson #B
Abilene, TX 79603

AIDS ARMS, Inc.
Office: (214) 521-5191
Fax: (214) 528-5891
4300 MacArthur
Suite 160
Lock Box 5
Dallas, TX 75209
Services Provided: Other, Non-HIV

AIDS Foundation of Houston
Hotline: (713) 524-2437
Office: (713) 623-6796
3202 Wesleyan Annex

Houston, TX 77027
Services Provided: Housing, Food, Care,
Info, Publish, Other

AIDS Interfaith Network
Office: (214) 559-4899
Fax: (214) 559-2465
4300 MacArthur
Suite 170
Dallas, TX 75219
Services Provided: Support, Care, Info,
Publish

AIDS Services of Austin
Hotline: (512) 451-2273
Post Office Box 4874
Austin, TX 78765

Blue Light Candle Project
Office: (210) 731-8430
Fax: (210) 731-8430
Post Office Box 12444
San Antonio, TX 78212
Services Provided: Info, Publish, Policy,
Sales, Other

City of Houston HIV/AIDS Hotline
Hotline: (713) 794-9092
8000 N. Stadium Drive
Houston, TX 77054

Coastal Bend AIDS Foundation
Hotline: (512) 814-7001
Office: (512) 814-2001
Fax: (512) 814-6502
Post Office Box 331416
527 Gordon Street
Corpus Christi, TX 78404
Services Provided: Support, Care, Info,
Publish, $, Other, Non-HIV

Dallas AIDS Resource Center
Hotline: (214) 559-2437
Office: (214) 521-5124

Fax: (214) 522-4604
2701 Reagan Street
Dallas, TX 75219
*Services Provided: Food, Info, Other,
Publish, Policy, $, Med*

Dallas County Health Department
AIDS Prevention Project
2377 N. Stemmons Freeway
Dallas, TX 75207-2710

Ector County Health Department
Permian Basin AIDS Resource Center
221 N. Texas Avenue
Odessa, TX 79761

El Paso City/County Health District
Office: (915) 543-3560
Fax: (915) 543-3566
Tillman Center
222 S. Campbell, #104
El Paso, TX 79901
*Services Provided: Med, Support, Info,
Pharm, Other, Non-HIV*

Fort Worth Counseling Center
AIDS Community Outreach
659 S. Jennings
Fort Worth, TX 76104

Harris County Health Department
Office: (713) 439-6000
Fax: (713) 439-6060
2223 W. Loop South
Houston, TX 77027
Services Provided: Info, Other, Non-HIV

Hispanic AIDS Committee
Office: (210) 227-2204
Fax: (210) 227-2205
814 Camden
San Antonio, TX 78215
*Services Provided: Support, Housing, Food,
Info, Publish, Other, Non-HIV*

Informa SIDA
Hotline: (512) 472-2001
1643 E. 2nd Street
Austin, TX 78702

Montrose Clinic
Hotline: (713) 520-2000
Office: (713) 520-2080
Fax: (713) 528-4923
215 Westheimer
Houston, TX 77006
*Services Provided: Med, Info, Pharm, Other,
Non-HIV*

Montrose Counseling Center
900 Lovett Boulevard, Suite 203
Houston, TX 77006

Panhandle AIDS Support Organization
Office: (806) 372-1050
604 W. 8th Street
Amarillo, TX 79101

Parkland Memorial Hospital
AIDS Clinic
5201 Harry Hines Boulevard
Dallas, TX 75235

People with AIDS Coalition/Houston
Office: (713) 522-5428
Fax: (713) 522-2674
1475 W. Gray
#163
Houston, TX 77019
*Services Provided: Support, Care, Info,
Publish, Other*

San Antonio AIDS Foundation
Hotline: (210) 225-4715
818 E. Grayson
San Antonio, TX 78208

South Plains AIDS Resource Center
Hotline: (806) 792-7783

Office: (806) 796-7068
Fax: (806) 796-0920
4204 B-50th
Post Office Box 6949
Lubbock, TX 79493
*Services Provided: Med, Support, $,
Housing, Food, Care, Info, Publish, Legal,
Pharm, Other*

Southwest AIDS Committee
Office: (915) 772-3366
1505 Mescalero Street
El Paso, TX 79925
*Services Provided: Support, Housing, Care,
Info, Legal, $, Med, Other*

Texas Department of Health
Texas AIDSLINE
Hotline: (512) 458-7400
1100 W. 49th Street
Austin, TX 78756

Triangle AIDS Network
Hotline: (409) 832-8338
Office: (409) 832-8338
Fax: (409) 832-0976
2544 Broadway
Post Office Box 12279
Beaumont, TX 77726
*Services Provided: Support, Housing, Food,
Care, Info, Publish, $, Other*

Valley AIDS Council
Hotline: (210) 428-9322
2220 Haine Drive
Suite 33
Harlingen, TX 78550

Utah

Day-to-Day HIV/AIDS Services
Office: (801) 944-4370
9863 S. Kramer Drive
Sandy, UT 84092

*Services Provided: Support, Housing, Care,
Info*

PWA Coalition of Utah
Office: (801) 484-2205
1390 S. 1100 E #107
Salt Lake City, UT 84105-2443
*Services Provided: Support, Info, Publish,
Other*

Utah AIDS Foundation
Hotline: (801) 487-2323
1408 S. 1100 E
Salt Lake City, UT 84105

Vermont

Vermont Cares
Hotline: (802) 863-2437
Post Office Box 5248
Burlington, VT 05402
*Services Provided: Support, Care, Info,
Publish, Legal, $*

Vermont CARES
38 Converse Court
Burlington, VT 05401

Vermont State Department of Health
The AIDS Program
Hotline: (802) 863-7245
Post Office Box 70
Burlington, VT 05402

Virgin Islands

Department of Health/Virgin Islands St.
    Thomas
HIV Project
Hotline: (809) 774-3168
St. Thomas Island, VI 802

Virginia

AIDS Council of Western Virginia
Hotline: (703) 982-AIDS
Office: (703) 985-0131
502 Campbell Avenue SW
Roanoke, VA 24004
Services Provided: Info, Publish, Other

AIDS Support Group
Post Office Box 2322
Charlottesville, VA 22902

Richmond AIDS Information Network
Hotline: (804) 358-2437
1721 Hanover Avenue
Richmond, VA 23220

Richmond AIDS Ministry (RAM)
Office: (804) 321-2170
Fax: (804) 321-6718
1005 W. Brookland Park Boulevard
#104
Richmond, VA 23220
*Services Provided: Support, Housing, Care,
Info, Publish, Legal*

Tidewater AIDS Crisis Task Force
Office: (804) 626-0127
Fax: (804) 627-4641
740 Duke Street
#520
Norfolk, VA 23510-1515
Services Provided: Support, Care, Info, Other

Virginia Department of Health
STD/AIDS Hotline
Hotline: (804) 533-4148
Office: (804) 225-4844
Fax: (804) 225-3517
Post Office Box 2448
Richmond, VA 23218
Services Provided: Info, Other, Non-HIV

Washington (State)

Kitsap County AIDS Task Force
109 Austin Drive
Bremerton, WA 98312

Northwest AIDS Foundation
Hotline: (206) 329-6923
127 Broadway East
Suite 200
Seattle, WA 98102-5711

People of Color against AIDS
Office: (206) 322-7061
Fax: (206) 322-7204
1200 S. Jackson
#25
Seattle, WA 98144
Services Provided: Info, Publish, Sales, Other

Seattle AIDS Support Group
Office: (206) 322-AIDS
Fax: (206) 322-2437
303 17th Avenue E
Seattle, WA 98112
Services Provided: Support, Info

Seattle Gay Clinic
Office: (206) 461-4540
500 19th Avenue East
Seattle, WA 98112
Services Provided: Med, Info

Shanti/Seattle
Office: (206) 322-0279
Post Office Box 20698
Seattle, WA 98102
Services Provided: Support, Care

Washington State HIV/AIDS Hotline
Department of Health Services—HIV/
AIDS
Hotline: (206) 586-0426

Post Office Box 47840
Olympia, WA 98504-7840

Washington, D.C.

Indochinese Community Center
AIDS Education Project
Office: (202) 462-4330
Fax: (202) 462-2774
1628 16th Street NW
Washington, DC 20009
*Services Provided: Support, Info, Publish,
Other*

Inner City AIDS Network
Office: (202) 543-6669
Fax: (202) 543-5364
813 L Street SE
Washington, DC 20002
Services Provided: Support, Info, Publish

Whitman-Walker Clinic
Hotline: (202) 332-AIDS
1407 S Street NW
Washington, DC 20009

West Virginia

AIDS Task Force of Upper Valley
Office: (304) 232-6295
Post Office Box 6360
Wheeling, WV 26003-6360
*Services Provided: Support, Care, Info,
Publish, Other*

Charleston AIDS Network
Post Office Box 1024
Charleston, WV 25324

Mountain State AIDS Network
Hotline: (304) 292-9000
235 High Street
#306
Morgantown, WV 26505

Ruby Memorial Hospital HIV Clinic
Hotline: (304) 293-3306
West Virginia University
Morgantown, WV 26506

Tri-State AIDS Task Force
Office: (304) 522-4357
824 Fifth Avenue
Suite 305
Huntington, WV 25704
*Services Provided: Med, Support, Housing,
Care, Info, Legal, Other*

Wisconsin

AIDS Resource Center of Wisconsin
Hotline: (414) 273-1991
315 W. Court Street
Milwaukee, WI 53212

Center Project, Inc.
824 S. Broadway
Green Bay, WI 54303

La Crosse County Health Department
AIDS/HIV Education Program
Office: (608) 785-9872
300 Fourth Street North
La Crosse, WI 54601

Madison AIDS Support Network
Post Office Box 731
Madison, WI 53701

Milwaukee AIDS Project
Hotline: (414) 273-2437
Office: (414) 273-1991
820 N. Plankinton
Milwaukee, WI 53203
*Services Provided: Support, Housing, Legal,
Food, $, Care, Info, Publish, Policy, Other*

Racine Health Department HIV Antibody
 Counseling and Testing

730 Washington Avenue
Racine, WI 53403

Southeast Wisconsin AIDS Project
6927 39th Avenue
Kenosha, WI 53141-0173

Wyoming

Wyoming AIDS Hotline
Hotline: (307) 777-5800
Hathaway Building
2300 Capitol Avenue, 4th Floor
Cheyenne, WY 82002-0710

Wyoming AIDS Project
Hotline: (307) 237-7833
Post Office Box 9353
Caspar, WY 82609

NON-HIV/AIDS RELATED

Alcoholics Anonymous
Hotline: (212) 870-3400
Fax: (212) 870-3003
475 Riverside Drive, 11th Floor
New York, NY 10115

Human Rights Campaign Fund
1012 14th Street NW, Suite 600
Washington, DC 20077-4462

March of Dimes
1275 Mamaroneck Avenue
White Plains, NY 10605

Narcotics Anonymous
World Service Office
Hotline: (818) 780-3951
Post Office Box 9999
Van Nuys, CA 91409

National Cocaine Hotline
Hotline: (800) 262-2463
Post Office Box 100
Summit, NJ 07902

PFLAG—Parents/Friends of Lesbians
    and Gays
Hotline: (212) 463-0629
Office: (212) 463-0629
Post Office Box 553
Lenox Hill Station
New York, NY 10021

California (Southern)
Gay and Lesbian Adolescent Social
    Services
650 N. Robertson Blvd.
Suite A
West Hollywood, CA 90069

Gay Men of Color
1169 N. Vermont Avenue
Los Angeles, CA 90029

Hemophilia Foundation
Hotline: (212) 682-5510
Office: (212) 682-5510
104 E. 40th Street
Suite 506
New York, NY 10016
*Services Provided: Support, Info, Publish, $,
Non-HIV*

Herpes Hotline
Hotline: (212) 213-6150
51 E. 25th Street, 6th Floor
New York, NY 10010

Hetrick-Martin Institute (for Gay and
    Lesbian Youth)
Hotline: (212) 674-2400
Fax: (212) 674-8650
2 Astor Place
New York, NY 10003

Lupus Foundation
Hotline: (212) 685-4118
149 Madison Avenue
Room 608
New York, NY 10016

National League for Nursing
350 Hudson Street
New York, NY 10014

SAGE (Senior Action in a Gay
    Environment)
Hotline: (212) 741-2247
208 W. 13th Street, 2nd Floor
New York, NY 10011

Sexually Transmitted Disease Hotline
Hotline: (212) 427-5120

158 E. 115th Street, 4th Floor
New York, NY 10029

International AFL-CIO, Department of
    Gay and Lesbian Services
Office: (202) 898-3443
AFL-CIO, CLC
1313 L Street NW
Washington, DC 20005
Services Provided: Info, Publish

U.S. Conference of Mayors
Office: (202) 293-7330
1620 I Street NW, 4th Floor
Washington, DC 20006

GLOSSARY OF TERMS

I am a Bear of Very Little Brain, and long words Bother me.
—*WINNIE-THE-POOH*
A. A. Milne

Like any other activity, industry, or hobby, living with HIV/AIDS has its own vocabulary of strange words, confusing abbreviations and acronyms, and even everyday words that are used to mean something different than they normally do.

Just like learning the native language before visiting a foreign country, it makes all the difference in the world to know the basics, even if it's impossible to know every word that you might come across.

What follows is a list of over three hundred of the most common, most confusing, or most important terms. Knowing these, you will be able to ask the right questions, and have a framework from which you can understand the answers.

For those who really like to do their homework, you might also seriously consider buying a large medical dictionary, the *Physician's Desk Reference* (a detailed description of all drugs), and a good book on human anatomy. Please see "Appendix A: Suggested Reading."

Often two or more words, brand names, scientific names, medical names, abbreviations, or acronyms are used to mean the same thing. In this case, the most common choice is listed first, with the other words listed in parentheses and cross-referenced. All glossary terms are in **bold type**, so that the reader may easily spot them and look them up elsewhere in the glossary.

Listings include a phonetic spelling in square brackets of unusual words, to help you pronounce them. Some abbreviations and acronyms are pronounced as if they were words. These have the phonetic spelling for that word in lower case, for example, AIDS [aides]. Other acronyms are spoken as letters spelled out, and these have their phonetic spelling as spaced out capital letters, for example, HIV [H I V].

I might not know how to use 34 words where three would do, but that does not mean I don't know what I'm talking about.
—RUTH SHAYS

A

absolute CD4 count: see **helper T-cells.**

acupressure or **acupuncture:** [ac-cue-pre-sure; ac-cue-punc-ture] A technique for healing and pain management developed by the ancient Chinese. Either strong pressure is applied (acupressure) or long, thin, needles are inserted and stimulated (acupuncture) at very specific points of the body.

acute: [a-cute] A condition that has come about quickly. The opposite of **chronic.**

acyclovir (brand name **Zovirax®**): [a-sy-cloe-vear] An antiviral drug used to treat **herpes.**

affirmation: [a-firm-ma-shun] A positive statement that is repeated, aloud or silently, over and over, to encourage self-healing, or self-image.

aggressive: [a-gres-sive] Referring to a treatment that may be very toxic, or have significant **side effects,** but that may be justified because it can get results quickly.

AIDS (acquired immune deficiency syndrome): [aides] AIDS is not actually a single disease itself, but a family of diseases and conditions that can occur after the immune system has been severely damaged. HIV is widely accepted as being the cause of this breakdown of the immune system, although some other factors in addition to HIV may well be involved or required.

A person is said to have AIDS if they are both HIV-**positive** and have *ever* had any AIDS-**defining condition.** The **CDC (Centers for Disease Control)** has published a list of conditions that qualify, most recently updated in 1993. These conditions are serious, life-challenging **infections** or **cancers** that people with normally healthy immune systems would be able to fight off. There are also some other conditions, such as a having a helper T-cell count below 200 that are on the CDC's AIDS-defining list.

   The **opportunistic diseases** that are made possible by the poorly functioning **immune system** are usually life-challenging, but often treatable, **chronic** conditions. Technically, people never die from AIDS itself, but rather from these opportunistic diseases.

   Once a person has met any AIDS-defining condition, he or she is defined as having AIDS for the rest of his or her life, regardless of his or her current level of health. Having AIDS, therefore, may say very little about that person's relative health, but it can say a lot about which government services, insurance, and other benefits he or she may qualify for.
(also see HIV; **opportunistic infections**; **AIDS-defining condition**; **helper T-cells**; and "Chapter 7: Becoming Your Own Medical Expert")

AIDS **dementia**: see **dementia**.

AIDS-**defining condition**: Any one of the twenty-five criteria that include certain **opportunistic infections** and other conditions, such as **wasting syndrome** or a **helper T-cell** count below 200, that are listed in the **CDC (Centers for Disease Control)** definition of who has, and who does not have AIDS. This definition was last updated in 1993. (also see AIDS; **opportunistic infections; candidiasis; cervical cancer; coccidioidomycosis; cryptococcosis; cryptosporidiosis, chronic; cytomegalovirus; encephalopathy; herpes simplex; histoplasmosis; isosporiasis; KS (Kaposi's sarcoma); lymphoma; MAI (mycobacterium avium intracellulare); mycobacterium tuberculosis; PCP (pneumocystis carinii pneumonia); pneumonia; progressive multifocal leukoencephalopathy; salmonella septicemia; TB (tuberculosis); toxoplasmosis; wasting syndrome** and "Chapter 7: Becoming Your Own Medical Expert")

AIDS-**related complex**: see **ARC**.

allergy: [al-ler-jee] An immune reaction caused by the presence of some foreign substance in the body. Common allergies include pollen, fur, feathers, insect venom, and various foods, chemicals, and drugs, although almost any substance can cause an allergy.

alpha interferon (brand name **Reoferon-A®**): [al-fa in-ter-fear-on]

An anticancer drug given by injection used to treat KS (Kaposi's sarcoma) and HIV **infection** itself.

alternative therapies: Non-Western medical techniques, often based on Chinese or folk medicine, that use natural or nontoxic methods to promote healing. Few alternative therapies have been given sufficient scientific study to determine which ones are effective and which ones are worthless. Although some of these may be miracle cures, many are undoubtedly merely quackery and outright fraud.

amphotericin B (brand name **Fungoizone IV®**): [am-fo-ter-i-sin] An antifungal drug that is often effective against most of the **fungi** that affect people with HIV.

anabolic steroids: [ann-a-bol-lick stair-roids] A treatment for **PCP**, although primarily known for their dangerous (and illegal) use by bodybuilders to increase muscle mass and weight.

analgesic: [ann-al-jee-sick] Any substance that reduces pain without causing unconsciousness.

anemia: [a-nee-mee-ya] A condition where there are too few red blood cells, too little hemoglobin, or too little blood in the body. Symptoms include fatigue, weakness, heart palpitations, dizziness, and exhaustion. Severe anemia can be corrected by transfusions. Anemia is a frequent **side effect** of many treatments.

anti-inflammatory: [ann-tea-in-flam-ma-tor-ree] Any substance that prevents or reduces inflammation.

antibacterial: [ann-tea-back-tear-e-al] Any substance that prevents or reduces the growth of bacteria.

antibiotic: [ann-tea-by-ot-ic] Any substance that prevents or reduces the growth of **microorganisms** such as **bacteria**, **fungi** and **parasites**, thus curing the conditions or diseases that these microorganisms cause.

antibodies: [ann-tea-bod-ees] Any substance which the body recognizes as foreign, such as **bacteria**, **fungi**, **parasites**, and **viruses**, is called an *antigen*. The **immune system** produces a protein called an *antibody* that is designed to help seek out and destroy or neutralize that unique type of *antigen*. This is the basis for all **immune response** in the body. Some antibodies make a person immune to a disease, while others do not.

antiemetic: [ann-tea-ah-met-ick] Any substance that prevents or reduces nausea and vomiting.

antifungal: [ann-tea-fun-gul] Any substance that prevents or reduces the growth of a **fungus**.

antigens: see **antibodies**

antiplacebo effect: [ann-tea pla-see-bow] The *placebo effect* is when an ineffective substance or treatment (like colored water or sugar pills) produces real, measurable results because the patient so strongly believed that it would. The *antiplacebo effect* is just the opposite: a scientifically proven effective substance or treatment is prevented from producing results because the patient so strongly believed that it would not work.

antiretroviral: see **antiviral**

antiviral: [ann-tea-vie-ral] Any substance that prevents or reduces the activity of a specific **virus** or stops that virus from reproducing. Often used as a shorthand for a treatment against the HIV virus itself. (also see **ddC; ddI; d4T; AZT (zidovudine)** and "Chapter 7: Becoming Your Own Medical Expert")

APLA (AIDS Project Los Angeles): Los Angeles–based, but an important national resource, APLA is the world's second-largest community-based AIDS service organization. (see "Appendix B: National and Regional Resources")

approved: A drug or other medical product that has been approved for marketing by the **Food and Drug Administration (FDA)** or a course of treatment that is considered acceptable by the American Medical Association (AMA).

ARC (AIDS-related complex): [ark] A term no longer generally used, and never officially recognized or defined by the **CDC (Centers for Disease Control)**. ARC describes a variety of HIV/AIDS-related symptoms or even serious illnesses that are not included in the definition of AIDS. Now referred to as **HIV-positive symptomatic**.

asymptomatic: [a-simp-toe-mat-ic] Without apparent significant symptoms but nonetheless experiencing some disease or condition. Sometimes used as a shortened form of **HIV-positive asymptomatic**.

atrophy: [at-tro-fee] A decrease in size or functionality, often as a result of being unused for prolonged time, hence the phrase "use it or lose it."

AZT (azidothymidine; zidovudine; brand name Retrovir®): Burroughs Wellcome, the drug manufacturer, makes zidovudine [zi-doe-view-dine] under the brand name of Retrovir®. AZT is the abbreviation of zidovudine's more technical chemical name, azidothymidine. AZT is used an antiviral treatment against the HIV **virus** itself, often in combination with other antiviral drugs. Although AZT is the oldest and the most widely accepted treatment against HIV, many believe that it can be ineffective at best, and highly toxic or even fatal at worst. There is strong, compelling evidence on *both sides* of this issue. (also see **antiviral** and "Chapter 7: Becoming Your Own Medical Expert")

B

B-cells (B-lymphocytes): One type of **white blood cell** that some believe to be produced in the **bone marrow**. B-cells produce **antibodies** to help fight or prevent disease.

bacteria: [back-tear-e-ya] Any of a certain group of microscopic organisms. Some bacteria can cause disease when they infect humans.

Bactrim®: [brand name **Septra®, trimethoprim/sulfamethoxazole, TMP/SMZ**] A drug used for **prophylaxis** (prevention) and treatment of **PCP (pneumocystis carinii pneumonia).**

baseline: A test result taken before treatment of a progressive disease, to which later measurements can be compared.

benign: [bee-nine] Not threatening health or life. Some tumors, for example, are benign.

beta-2 microglobulin: [bay-ta two mi-crow-glob-you-lin] A protein found in the blood. Elevated levels of beta-2 microglobulin may indicate replication or progression of HIV.

biopsy: [by-op-see] Surgical removal and laboratory testing of **tissue** from the living body, often providing the most accurate diagnosis of a disease or condition.

blood pressure: A measurement of the force with which blood presses against the sides of a blood vessel. The pressure is measured at two points: when the heart is contracting (systolic pressure) and when the heart is between contractions (diastolic pressure). In healthy young people, the systolic reading is typically 100 to 140; the diastolic reading is typically 60 to 90. This is written as systolic over diastolic, for example "120/80."

blood type: A method of classifying blood according to the presence or absence of certain genetically determined proteins in the **red blood cells** that make some types of blood incompatible with others for transfusions. There are four general classifications: Type A, Type B, Type AB and Type O, each of which may be Rh factor positive or negative, thus giving eight major blood types.

blood work: Diagnostic laboratory tests measuring various properties of the blood, often including **T-cells**, and other indicators of health.

body fluids: Any fluid manufactured within the body. In terms of HIV/ AIDS, this is often used as a shorthand for semen, blood, vaginal lu-brication, and breast milk, the four body fluids that can cause HIV **infection**. Other body fluids, such as saliva, sweat, vomit, etc. are not able to transmit HIV, although they could also contain blood, which can cause HIV transmission.

bone marrow: [bone mar-row] The spongelike **tissue** located in the hollow center of many bones where certain blood cells are formed. Bone marrow can be withdrawn (by placing a needle in the hipbone) and analyzed to detect abnormalities in blood cell production.

bronchoscopy: [bron-ko-sco-pee] A diagnostic procedure for looking at the lungs with flexible fiber optics. Often used as a diagnostic tool for PCP.

buyers club: A group that sells *"underground drugs"* to people with HIV/ AIDS, usually for little or no profit. These drugs have not yet been approved for use in the U.S. by the **Food and Drug Administration** (and are therefore not technically legal). Unfortunately, since these drugs have not been fully tested nor is the quality carefully monitored, they may well be useless or even toxic. (also see **alternative therapies**)

C

cancer: [can-sir] A large group of diseases characterized by uncontrolled growth and spread of abnormal cells. The three cancers associated with HIV/AIDS are **lymphoma**, **KS**, and **cervical cancer** in women.

candidiasis: [can-di-di-a-sis] *Candida albicansis* is a yeastlike **fungus** that is common in the general population affecting the mouth, skin, intestinal tract, and vagina. Normally, the **immune system** can keep the growth of this fungus under control. Candidiasis occurs when this candida **infection** takes hold. In the mouth and throat it is also called **thrush**, and in the vagina it is also called a yeast infection. Thrush is extremely common in people with HIV infection. In those who have weakened immune systems, candidiasis can become **chronic**, extremely painful, and even potentially dangerous. Some chronic forms can be an AIDS-**defining condition**.

carcinoma: [car-sin-om-a] A **malignant** tumor or **cancer** that may spread to other parts of the body.

CAT scan: see **CT Scan.**

catheter: [cath-e-ter] A surgically implanted tube entering the skin on the chest and leading to a large vein. Rather than inject a person many times each day over a long period to administer **intravenous** drug therapy, a **Hickman catheter** is left in place and can easily and painlessly be connected for **infusion** of medication.

CBC (complete blood count): A specific blood test that analyzes cell counts, **hematocrit**, and hemoglobin cell volume.

cc (ml, cubic centimeter): A unit of liquid measure, also called a milliliter, or 1/1000 of a **liter**. Approximately equal to 1/5 of a teaspoon.

CDC (Centers for Disease Control): A federal agency that is a branch of the Public Health Service providing public health resources for state and local health departments. The CDC provides national health and safety guidelines, **epidemiology**, disease tracking, and statistical data on HIV/AIDS as well as all other communicable diseases and other threats to the public health.

cerebral: Relating to the brain.

cervical cancer: see AIDS-**defining condition** and "Chapter 7: Becoming Your Own Medical Expert."

chemotherapy: [kee-mo-ther-a-pee] The use of aggressive chemical agents in the treatment of disease, usually **cancer**.

chlamydia: [cla-mid-e-ya] A **microorganism** which causes **infections** in the eye, urethra, and a variety of other symptoms. Chlamydia is an

STD (sexually transmitted disease) independent of AIDS, but it can also appear as an HIV/AIDS-related opportunistic infection.

chronic: [kron-nick] Continuous, persistent, or long-term. The opposite of acute.

clinical: Based on observation of actual patients and their symptoms.

clinical trial: A scientifically controlled test to see how well a new drug works on actual patients. See phase-I, phase-II, and phase-III trials.

CMV (cytomegalovirus): [sy-toe-meg-ah-lo-vi-rus] The CMV virus, a member of the herpes family, is commonly found in people without HIV infection. Usually the immune system holds CMV in check, and CMV remains dormant in the body without causing any serious disease. With a severely weakened immune system it can become serious, particularly when affecting the retina of the eye, which if left untreated, can cause blindness. (also see AIDS-defining condition and "Chapter 7: Becoming Your Own Medical Expert")

cofactor: Any other condition, factor, or individual characteristic that may influence the progression of a disease or the likelihood of becoming ill, for example the presence of some chemical substance, microorganism, or a person's age, race, or genetic makeup. Currently, although HIV is the only proven cause of AIDS, there are probably other cofactors, such as other infections or behavior patterns that could expedite the progression to AIDS.

cold sore (fever blister): A herpes simplex infection of the lips or face. (also see herpes)

colon (large intestine or large bowel): The gastrointestinal tract begins at the mouth, continues down the esophagus, and is followed by (in order) the stomach, small intestine, colon, and, finally, the rectum.

colonoscopy: Visual examination of the colon using a special camera through a long flexible tube inserted in the anus.

combination therapy: The use of two or more drugs or types of treatment working together, to achieve better results than either could separately. (also see synergy)

community-based clinical trial (CBCT): A method of drug testing conducted by primary-care physicians in close cooperation with patients and AIDS advocates.

community-based organization: A local organization or agency that provides services to people with HIV/AIDS, such as New York's **GMHC (Gay Men's Health Crisis)**, Los Angeles' **APLA (AIDS Project Los Angeles)**, the various **Shanti projects, San Francisco AIDS Foundation**, Washington DC's **Whitman-Walker Clinic**. See "Appendix B: National and Regional Resources" for a partial listing, or in "Appendix A: Suggested Reading," under *Directories* refer to United States Conference of Mayors "Local AIDS Services: The National Directory," March 1994.

compassionate use: Prior to final testing and FDA approval, drug companies often donate quantities of a drug for free (since it would be generally illegal for them to sell it before approval) to people who have an urgent need for this new drug and would otherwise be unable to obtain it.

contagious: [con-tay-jus] Any infectious disease capable of being transmitted by casual contact from one person to another. HIV is not contagious since it can be transmitted only via direct or intimate contact.

contraindication: [con-tra-in-di-ca-shon] A condition, symptom, or other circumstance under which a drug or other treatment could be inadvisable or could be harmful. For example, many drugs are contraindicated for pregnant or nursing women. (also see **indication**)

control group: To be able to study the effectiveness of a drug, medical treatment, or anything else that affects a person (such as eating a low-fat diet) researchers compare a *test group* of people who do the thing that researchers are studying with a *control group* who do not, but in all other ways are the same. In "randomized" or "double-blind" trials, neither the researchers nor the participants know during the test who is in the *test group* getting actual drugs and who is in the *control group* getting a **placebo**, such as sugar pills.

cryptococcosis: [crip-toe-cock-coe-sis] *Cryptococcus neoformans* is a **fungus** that is usually acquired via the respiratory tract. Normally, the **immune system** can keep this under control. Cryptococcosis occurs when this fungal **infection** takes hold, often spreading to the meninges (the lining around the brain and spinal cord) and causing various neurological symptoms. (also see AIDS-**defining condition** and "Chapter 7: Becoming Your Own Medical Expert")

cryptosporidiosis: *Cryptosporidium* is a protozoan **parasite** found in the intestines of infected animals (including humans), and is usually acquired via direct contact with these animals or by eating contaminated food or water. Normally, the immune system can keep this under control. Cryptosporidiosis occurs when parasitic **infection** takes hold. In those who have weakened **immune systems**, cryptosporidiosis can become **chronic**, symptoms may include ongoing, profuse watery diarrhea, fever, and substantial weight loss. (also see AIDS-**defining condition** and "Chapter 7: Becoming Your Own Medical Expert")

CT Scan (computerized tomography scan): A diagnostic technique that builds a three-dimensional computer image of the body out of many two-dimensional X-ray views. Diagnostic techniques of this sort that do not require surgery and that have no ill effects are called "noninvasive." (also see **MRI**)

culture: [cul-ture] The growth of **microorganisms** or living **tissue** in the laboratory, in a gel, solution, or other medium that promotes their growth. Also the product of a good upbringing including frequent exposure to music, the arts, and fine food.

cytomegalovirus: see **CMV**.

Cytovene®: see **ganciclovir**.

D

d4T (stavudine, brand name Zerit®): An **antiviral** drug, similar in action to **AZT**, manufactured by Bristol-Myers Squibb, used to fight the HIV virus itself (also see **AZT**; **antiviral** and "Chapter 7: Becoming Your Own Medical Expert")

dapsone: [dap-sone] A drug used for **prophylaxis** (prevention) and treatment of **PCP (pneumocystis carinii pneumonia)**.

ddC (zalcitabine, brand name Hivid®): An **antiviral** drug, similar in action to AZT, manufactured by Hoffman-LaRoche under the brand name of Hivid® used to fight the HIV virus itself (also see **AZT**; **antiviral** and "Chapter 7: Becoming Your Own Medical Expert")

ddI (didanosine, brand name Videx®): An **antiviral** drug, similar in action to AZT, manufactured by Bristol-Myers Squibb under the brand name of Videx® used to fight the HIV virus itself (also see **AZT**; **antiviral** and "Chapter 7: Becoming Your Own Medical Expert")

dehydration: [de-high-dray-shon] The human body is over 80% water, and all of the reactions necessary for life use water, particularly for cleansing the body of waste and toxins. Dehydration occurs when there is not enough water for these processes. This can result from difficulty swallowing, lack of thirst, diarrhea, fatigue, or many other factors. Although each person's needs are different, a good rule of thumb is that every day, each person should drink at least 64 ounces of water, which is the same as about 8 large glasses, or about 2 liter or quart bottles.

dementia: [di-men-sha] The **chronic** loss of former mental capacity, memory, judgment, concentration, and emotional ability resulting from some physical cause. AIDS dementia can be caused by a number of factors, including the direct effect of HIV in the brain. AIDS-related dementia is only common in the very later stages of AIDS.

depression: [de-presh-on] The ongoing mental state of feeling unhappy, hopeless, discouraged, worthless, fatigued, and/or the loss of interest in pleasurable things. Symptoms include significant weight loss or gain, insomnia or excessive sleep, or other compulsive behaviors. AIDS-related depression is quite common, and can generally be treated by counseling or drug therapies.

dermatitis: [derm-a-ti-tis] An inflammation of the skin, such as a rash.

diagnosis: [die-ag-no-sis] An official, medical evaluation, often based on laboratory tests, that confirms the presence of a specific disease or other condition.

didanosine: see **ddI**.

Diflucan®: see **fluconazole**.

disseminated: [dis-sem-min-ate-ted] Scattered throughout the body.

double-blind clinical trial: In order to prove statistically the effectiveness of a drug, neither the administering doctors nor the experimental subjects know during the test who is in the *test group* getting a test drug and who is in the *control group* getting a **placebo**, such as sugar pills. Although this form of testing provides the most meaningful statistical information, many people feel that it is more important to provide treatments that *seem* promising to those who urgently need them, regardless of the potential risks, rather than wait for statistically definitive proof.

drug resistance: The ability of a disease-causing organism, **microor-**

ganism, or virus to be unaffected by drugs that usually cure or control that disease.

E

efficacy: [ef-fik-a-see] The ability of a treatment to produce the desired effect.

electrolyte: [e-lek-tro-lite] The dissolved salts found in blood, **tissue,** fluids, and cells.

ELISA (enzyme linked immunosorbent assay): [eh-lie-za] A blood test that detects **antibodies** to certain **microorganisms,** including HIV. Some forms of this test can deliver extremely accurate results within fifteen minutes. The ELISA test is very sensitive, meaning that if HIV **antibodies** are present, the test result will be positive; however, it is not very precise, meaning that the test will be *falsely* positive because of other antibodies. Because of this, a positive result must then be followed by a confirmatory test such as the **Western Blot** test (which may takes many days or even weeks) to distinguish whether these are HIV antibodies or from some other cause. A negative result, on the other hand, does not completely prove that someone has not been infected with the HIV **virus,** since it may take as long as six months to develop enough HIV antibodies to be detected.

encephalitis: [in-sef-a-lie-tis] An **infection** or inflammation of the brain, usually caused by a **virus** but sometimes by bacteria. Similar to meningitis, an infection of the meninges, the membrane surrounding the brain and spinal cord. (also see **encephalopathy**)

encephalopathy: [in-sef-a-lop-a-thee] Any disease of the brain, particularly one in which the actual structure of the brain becomes changed. (also see AIDS-**defining condition; encephalitis;** and "Chapter 7: Becoming Your Own Medical Expert")

endoscopy: A diagnostic procedure to examine an internal organ or body cavity without surgery by passing a flexible fiber-optic cable through the mouth or rectum.

epidemic: [epi-dem-ic] Many more cases of a disease than would normally be expected.

epidemiology: [epi-dee-mi-o-lo-jee] The scientific study of epidemics, particularly to determine the specific causes, monitor the extent, recommend treatments, and prevent future outbreaks.

Epstein-Barr virus (EBV): [ep-steen bar] Epstein-Barr is a herpeslike **virus** that is contagious, infects the nose and throat, and can lie dormant in the lymph glands for many years. It is widely recognized as the cause of infectious mononucleosis (mono). (also see **mononucleosis**)

esophagus: [eh-sof-a-gus] The muscular tube that connects the throat to the stomach.

euthanasia: [youth-in-asia] The process of allowing or causing a terminally ill person to die. A highly controversial subject, addressed in "Chapter 10: Simplifying and Reevaluating Life and Death." Many people consider euthanasia to be the most humane, compassionate alternative for someone who would otherwise linger in great pain; other people consider it to be either murder or suicide, and, therefore, morally wrong in any circumstances.

exclusion criteria: see **inclusion criteria**.

expanded access (open label study): A step just before approval of a new drug by the FDA, where people who are not participating in the **clinical trials** may be able to receive the drug from the manufacturer.

experimental drug: A drug that is still in the testing phase prior to approval by the FDA. Since testing is not complete, beneficial and harmful effects and the most-effective dosages may not yet be known.

F

false negative: A test result that indicates the absence of an **infection** or other condition, when in fact it is present. Often used as shorthand to mean "incorrectly diagnosed as HIV negative." This is usually the result of someone being tested in the "**window period**" (can be as long as six months) between infection and the body producing enough **antibodies** to be testable. (also see "Chapter 7: Becoming Your Own Medical Expert")

false positive: A test result that indicates the presence of an **infection** or other condition, when in fact there is none. Often used as shorthand to mean "incorrectly diagnosed as HIV-positive." The combination of the **ELISA** test and **Western Blot** are extremely accurate, with considerably less than a one-percent error rate. However, any test result can be incorrect, and should be repeated if necessary.

flu: see **influenza.**

fluconazole (brand name **Diflucan**®): [flu-con-ah-zole] An **antifungal** drug manufactured by Pfizer Pharmaceuticals.

Food and Drug Administration (FDA): The U.S. federal agency that is responsible for the testing and regulation of drugs.

Fungoizone IV®: see **amphotericin B.**

fungus, fungi: [fun-gus, fun-guy] A type of **microbe** (microscopic plant) that includes mushrooms, yeast, and molds. **Fungi** (the plural of fungus) cause **infections** such as **thrush,** cryptococcal meningitis, and **PCP.**

G

ganciclovir (brand name **Cytovene**®): [gan-sy-clo-vir] An **intravenous antiviral** drug used to treat **CMV (cytomegalovirus), herpes simplex,** and other **viruses.**

generic drugs: [jen-air-ik drugs] Generic drugs are lower-priced alternatives that are chemically equivalent to brand names. For example *Tylenol*® is the brand name used by the Johnson & Johnson company for tablets containing the *generic* drug acetaminophen. Other companies may sell very similar acetaminophen tablets, so long as it is clear that these are not *Tylenol*® brand acetaminophen. Many doctors prefer to prescribe generic drugs rather than brand names so that their patients buy the least-expensive choice that is chemically identical. Many drug companies claim that generic drugs are not necessarily of the same high quality as their brand.

genitals: Sexual organs.

GMHC (Gay Men's Health Crisis): New York-based, but an important national resource, GMHC is the world's oldest and largest community-based AIDS service organization. (also see "Appendix B: National and Regional Resources")

gonorrhea: [gone-a-re-ah] A common sexually transmitted disease that is caused by a bacterium, and can be cured by **antibiotics.**

H

hairy leukoplakia: see **leukoplakia**.

half-life: The time it takes for half of the amount of some drug to be eliminated from the body. Since the less of a drug that is in the body, the more slowly it is eliminated from the body, in twice the half-life, ¾ of a drug will be eliminated from the body, the original half plus only half of the remaining half.

health maintenance organization (HMO): A health-care system where people or their employer pay a fixed fee for more or less unlimited health care, but must use "member" physicians and facilities.

helper T-cells (T4-lymphocytes, CD4): One of the many types of **white blood cells** that plays an important role in the **immune system**. Helper T-cells are able to detect foreign invaders in the body and they are essential for activating **antibody** production, **killer T-cells**, and other **immune responses**. By an unhappy accident, these are also the main cells that the HIV **virus** infects.

The number of T4 helper cells in every milliliter of blood is often used as an approximate indicator of the health of the immune system. Although this is widely accepted as one of the few measures of the health of someone's immune system, many other day-to-day factors can significantly affect these test results. Rather than look at any one test, one needs to look at a trend from many tests over a period of say six months or longer.

The normal range of T4 helper cells is about 500–1,000, counts of 200–400 are considered low, but not too alarming, and counts below 200 in people with HIV are now defined by the **CDC** as indicating AIDS, and are frequently advised to take steps against developing **opportunistic infections**. (also see HIV and "Chapter 7: Becoming Your Own Medical Expert")

hematocrit: [he-mat-oh-crit] The percentage of **red blood cells** as part of the total blood volume.

hemophilia: [he-moe-feel-ya] An inherited disease that almost exclusively affects males. A person with hemophilia does not produce an important protein that helps the blood to clot, and therefore will bleed easily unless he receives regular transfusions of clotting factor, which is produced from human blood. Before the blood supply was adequately safeguarded, many hemophiliacs became infected with HIV. (also see "Chapter 7: Becoming Your Own Medical Expert," regarding the blood supply)

hepatitis: [hep-a-tight-us] An inflammation of the **liver** caused by one of the hepatitis viruses. Often people do not have any symptoms and therefore do not even know they have it. Some people may experience fever, enlargement of the liver, or a yellow discoloration of the skin and eyes, which is called jaundice. Hepatitis B virus can be transmitted by sexual contact, contaminated needles or blood products and can be prevented by the Hepatitis B **vaccine**.

herpes: [her-peas] Herpes is both a family of diseases, as well as a family of **viruses** that causes these diseases. They can remain inactive or dormant in the body for years, and become reactivated by stress, trauma, other **infections**, or suppression of the **immune system**. (also see **herpes simplex; herpes zoster**)

herpes simplex: [her-peas sim-plex] Herpes simplex affects the mucous membranes and causes cold sores or fever blisters and painful sores on the anus and genitals, and can be transmitted through direct contact with an infected area. Chronic herpes simplex may be an AIDS-**defining condition** (also see **herpes; herpes zoster** and "Chapter 7: Becoming Your Own Medical Expert")

herpes zoster (shingles): [her-peas zos-ter] Herpes zoster is caused by the same **virus** as chicken pox and can reappear in adulthood to create painful blisters which are generally dry and itchy and may even leave minor scarring anywhere on the skin in a pattern that follows major nerve pathways. (also see **herpes; herpes simplex**)

Hickman catheter: [hick-man cath-e-ter] see **catheter**.

higher-risk behaviors: Any activity that has a "higher" likelihood of transmitting the HIV **virus** to another person, including sharing injection drug equipment, any type of unprotected (without a condom) sex with insertion (oral, anal, or vaginal) between either men or women who are either heterosexual, homosexual, or bisexual.

higher-risk groups: Originally used to describe those groups first affected by HIV/AIDS: gay and bisexual men, **injection drug users**, hemophiliacs, and the sexual partners of any in these groups. The term is no longer generally used because it implies that people outside of these groups are less likely to become HIV infected. This is not true:

there are no higher-risk groups, only **higher-risk behaviors**.

HIV (human immunodeficiency virus): [H I V] HIV is widely accepted as the virus that causes AIDS, although some other factor or factors may well be involved or required. Technically, HIV is a group of **retroviruses**, primarily HIV-1, that infect and destroy one of the key components of the human **immune system**, the helper T **white blood cells**.

HIV can only be transmitted from one person to another during an activity that can put HIV-infected blood, semen (cum), vaginal lubrication, or breast milk inside of another person.

Once exposed to air, HIV is destroyed in a few seconds. Unlike other viruses, HIV cannot be transmitted through any indirect or casual contact. HIV **infection** is not possible through other body fluids, such as saliva, tears, sweat, urine, vomit, or fecal matter, although any of these body fluids could also contain small amounts of blood that could carry HIV infection. In the fifteen-plus-year documented history of HIV/AIDS, there has not been one single known case of HIV infection through casual contact, even in the most extreme cases, such as those living with and caring for those with AIDS.

The credit for isolating the HIV virus is shared between Luc Montagnier of the Pasteur Institute in France who called it **LAV (Lymphadenopathy Associated Virus)** and by Robert Gallo of the National Institutes of Health in the United States who called it **HTLV-III (Human T-Lymphotophic Virus Type III).**

The most frequent (but not the only) means of HIV infection are unprotected vaginal sex, unprotected anal sex, or sharing injection drug equipment such as needles. (also see "Chapter 7: Becoming Your Own Medical Expert")

HIV-negative (HIV-): Testing negative for the presence of the HIV virus. A person who is HIV-negative might, in fact, be in the "**window period**" (which can be as long as six months), and therefore be so recently infected with the HIV virus that he or she is not yet producing enough **antibodies** to be testable. (also see "Chapter 7: Becoming Your Own Medical Expert")

HIV-positive (HIV+): Testing positive for the presence of the HIV virus. A person who is HIV-positive might not also have AIDS, and might never get AIDS. (also see HIV **virus** and AIDS)

HIV-positive asymptomatic: [HIV-positive a-sim-toe-matic] Being infected with the HIV **virus** (HIV-positive), but without any apparent significant symptoms.

HIV-positive symptomatic: [HIV-positive sim-toe-matic] Experiencing the symptoms, perhaps even significant symptoms, without being defined as having AIDS. Formerly called **ARC** (**AIDS-related complex**).

hives: [hives] An allergic reaction to drugs, certain foods, or stress that appears on the skin as patchy, itchy, raised areas.

Hivid®: see **ddC**.

holistic treatments: [holl-is-tik treet-ments] A type of treatment that focuses on increasing the health of a person as a whole, rather than merely curing isolated diseases or symptoms. (also see **alternative therapies**)

homophobia: [hoe-moe-phoe-bee-a] A moral judgment, emotional bias, fear, or prejudice against homosexuals.

host: The cell or organism that supports the growth of a **parasite** or **virus**.

HTLV-III (Human T-Lymphotophic Virus Type III): see **HIV**.

hyper: [hi-per] A prefix meaning above normal. Confusingly, this is the opposite of **hypo**, meaning below normal.

hypersensitivity: Greater than normal sensitivity or response to drugs or other substances.

hypo: [hi-po] A prefix meaning below normal. Confusingly, this is the opposite of **hyper**, meaning above normal.

I

idiopathic: [id-ee-o-path-ik] Without apparent or known cause.

IDU: Injection drug users.

immune deficiency: A reduction in the ability of the **immune system** to function properly, thus making someone unable to fight off diseases that they would not normally develop. (also see "Chapter 7: Becoming Your Own Medical Expert")

immune modulators: [im-yoon mod-you-late-ors] Any treatment or substance that increases or enhances the **immune system**, or stimulates the production of immune system cells.

immune response: The body's reaction to the presence of recognized foreign substances.

immune system: The body's own automatic way of fighting off disease and repairing itself when injured. The immune system is actually made up of a very complex interaction between the central nervous system (including the brain), various blood cells, internal organs, as well as internally produced hormones and other chemicals. The immune system recognizes foreign invaders, neutralizes them, and sometimes can remember that response later and mount a quicker defense when confronted with the same challenge.

immuno: [im-yoo-know] Pertaining to the **immune system**.

immunology: [im-yoo-nol-lo-jee] The branch of medicine that studies and treats diseases that involve the **immune system**.

in vitro: [in vee-tro] Studies conducted in the test tube, as opposed to studies conducted in humans or other living beings.

in vivo: [in vee-vo] Studies conducted in humans or other living beings, as opposed to studies conducted in the test tube.

inclusion criteria: [in-cloo-zhun cry-teer-ee-a] During a **clinical trial**, the rules that define who can be involved with the trial; for example, some trials may be open only to HIV-**positive** men who are not taking AZT and have greater than 500 T-cells.

incubation period: see **window period**.

indication: [in-dik-ay-shun] The diseases or conditions for which a drug or other course of treatment is officially recognized or recommended. For example, **Bactrim®** is indicated for PCP. (also see **contraindication**)

infection: [in-fek-shun] An infection occurs when a **virus**, bacterium, toxin, or other **microorganism** invades a part of the body in sufficient quantities to take hold and multiplies in sufficient quantities to take hold, survive, and cause disease.

influenza (flu): [in-floo-en-zuh] A disease caused by any member of the myxovirus family. Influenza is contagious and infects the mucous membranes and respiratory tract. Symptoms often include fever, chills, cough, sore throat, exhaustion, and muscle pain. Because there are so many subtly different types or strains of influenza, each year a new influenza **vaccine** is created to combat the anticipated strains for that year. Naturally, some years' vaccines are more effective than others, depending on how successful the vaccine makers were at predicting the strains of virus.

informed consent: A form of consumer protection. Before a patient is given some test, procedure, or starts an experimental program, they must sign a legal document stating that they have been given an explanation of all the important facts about this procedure, that they are able fully to understand these facts, and (most importantly) that after making a sound judgment based on these facts, they wish this procedure performed.

infusion: [in-fyoo-zhun] Injecting a liquid into the bloodstream, often to administer drugs, food, or other nutrients. This can be done once, or continued over many hours, days, or longer.

Injection drug users (IDU, Intravenous drug users, IVDU): People who share injection drug equipment, even **steroid** users, can transmit the HIV **virus**. Most people who use drugs do NOT consider themselves to be "drug addicts." Even onetime injection drug users can become HIV infected.

interaction: [in-ter-ak-shun] Often taking one drug will have a significant effect on the effectiveness of another drug. This interaction may increase the effect of one or both drugs, decrease the effect of one or both drugs, or cause serious **side effects** (also see **synergy**)

intramuscular injections: The injecting of drugs into the muscle **tissue** for slower absorption, rather than directly into the veins.

intravenous (IV): The injecting of drugs directly into the veins.

isosporiasis: see AIDS-**defining condition** and "Chapter 7: Becoming Your Own Medical Expert."

K

kg (kilogram): A measure of weight defined as 1000 grams, equal to 2.2046 pounds.

killer T-cells (killer T-lymphocytes): One of the many types of **white blood cells** that plays an important role in the **immune system**. After being alerted by the **helper T-cells**, the killer T-cells attach themselves to and kill foreign organisms.

KS (Kaposi's sarcoma): [Ca-po-see sar-co-ma] A form of malignant cancer which generally only affects people with weakened immune systems. KS is an AIDS-defining condition, and appears as soft pink, purple, blue, or brown spots on the skin. These can range from the size of a pea to a pancake, and are slightly raised, generally painless, and somewhat hard to the touch. Many people with external KS thrive for years. Eventually KS may spread to the lymph nodes and internal organs where it can become seriously life-challenging. (also see AIDS-defining condition and "Chapter 7: Becoming Your Own Medical Expert")

L

large intestine: see colon.

latency (dormancy): [late-en-see] The period when an organism is in the body but not actively reproducing or producing any ill effects.

LAV (Lymphadenopathy Associated Virus): see HIV.

lesion: [lee-zhun] An eruption on any patch of skin or other tissue that is abnormal due to injury or disease. Often used to describe the area affected by KS (Kaposi's sarcoma) or herpes.

leukocytes: see white blood cells.

leukopenia: [lew-koe-peen-e-ya] A low number (or *penia*) of white blood cells (or leukocytes), the cells of the immune system that fight infection. Do not confuse with leukoplakia.

leukoplakia: [lew-koe-play-key-a] Leukoplakia literally means "white patches," which generally occur in the mouth, where they are also called oral hairy leukoplakia (OHL). Leukoplakia produces few symptoms other than distorting taste and causing mild pain. It is thought to be related to the Epstein-Barr virus.

liter: [lee-ter] A measure of volume, equal to 33.8 liquid ounces or just under 4 1/4 cups or just over 1 quart.

lumbar puncture (spinal tap): [lum-bar punk-chur] A procedure where a small amount of spinal fluid is removed from the spinal column by a needle for testing.

lymph glands (lymph nodes): [limf nodz] Tiny organs distributed widely throughout the body that filter the lymph fluid and are involved with the **immune system**.

lymph: [limf] A clear or light yellow liquid, basically blood without the **red blood cells (plasma)**, that seeps outside of the blood vessels, and that flows through the lymphatic channels, ducts, and glands.

lymphadenopathy: [lim-fad-den-op-a-thee] A swelling, firmness, and possibly tenderness of the **lymph** nodes (glands). This may be caused by the HIV **virus** itself, some other **infection** such as the **influenza (flu)** or **mononucleosis (mono),** or from **lymphoma (cancer** of the lymph nodes). The medical term **persistent generalized lymphadenopathy (PGL)** is defined as having swollen lymph nodes for at least one month in two different sites of the body, not counting the groin area. Alone, there is very little predictive value in gauging one's current or future health based on the size of the lymph nodes.

lymphocytes: [lim-fo-sites] A subcategory of **white blood cells (leukocytes)** that include T-cells and B-cells (also see **red blood cells, T-cells, B cells)**

lymphoma: [lim-fo-ma] One of many forms of **cancer** of the lymphatic system (**lymph** nodes). Symptoms often include chronic lymph node swelling and extreme weight loss, sometimes accompanied by a fever. (also see AIDS-**defining condition** and "Chapter 7: Becoming Your Own Medical Expert")

M

MAC (mycobacterium avium complex): [my-co-back-tear-re-um] One of a family of diseases caused by an infection from the bacteria *mycobacterium avium,* which is related to the bacteria that causes tuberculosis. One of the most common is **MAI (mycobacterium avium intercellulare)** which spreads throughout the body causing cavities, such as the lungs, muscle, brain, skin, bones, to become filled with a cheesy material. About half of all people with AIDS are found to have MAI at the time of their death.

macrophage: [mak-ro-fayj] The **white blood cell** that specializes in surrounding and "eating" harmful matter in the blood system, particularly **bacteria**.

MAI (mycobacterium avium intercellulare): see **MAC.**

maintenance therapy: A treatment to maintain a desired effect once it has already been achieved.

malabsorption (intestinal malabsorption): [mal-ab-sorb-shun] Eating food or taking vitamins or drugs does not necessarily make them available for the body to be used. They must be digested and absorbed into the bloodstream, usually in the small intestine. Unfortunately, many factors can interfere with the effectiveness of the intestines in absorbing nutrients. In extreme cases without medical intervention, one could eat all day and still starve to death because the nutrient value in the food was passing right through the intestines without ever being available to the body.

malaise: [may-layz] A generalized, nonspecific feeling of discomfort or uneasiness.

malignant: [mal-lig-nant] A tumor or growth that is not contained in one area, but is growing and spreading out of control.

Marinol® (dronabinol): [mar-i-nol] The brand name of dronabinol, a synthetic version of tetra-hydrocannabinol, the active chemical in marijuana, used to reduce nausea and increase appetite in people with AIDS.

mechanical ventilation: When a person is unable to breathe on his or her own, a machine is used to keep that person breathing.

Medicaid: [med-i-kayd] A government program that provides medical care to the poor.

Medicare: [med-i-kayr] A government administered health insurance program for those aged sixty-five and over, providing some of the cost of hospitalization, inpatient services, and home care. Supplementary Medical Insurance is available for an additional fee.

meningitis: [men-in-ji-tis] An **infection** or inflammation of the meninges, the membranes that surround the brain and spinal cord. Meningitis may be caused by bacterial or viral infections; however, in people with HIV it is usually caused by *cryptococcosis meningitis*. Similar to *encephalitis*, which is an infection of the brain itself.

methadone: [meth-a-done] A prescription narcotic drug that is used as a substitute for morphine or heroin, although it is almost as addictive as the drugs it is replacing.

mg (milligram): A very small unit of measure of weight defined as

...ooo of a gram. There are about 28,350 milligrams in one ounce.

...robes: see microorganisms.

...icroorganisms (microbes): Very small organisms, such as **bacteria**, protozoa, **parasites**, **viruses**, and **fungi**, that are so small they require a microscope to be seen.

mononucleosis (mono): [mon-o-noo-clee-o-sis] **Epstein-Barr** is a herpeslike virus that is contagious, infects the nose and throat, and can lie dormant in the **lymph glands** for many years. It is widely recognized as the cause of infectious mononucleosis (mono).

MRI (magnetic resonance imaging): A diagnostic technique that produces three-dimensional computer images of the internal organs and **tissue** inside the body without surgery. Diagnostic techniques of this sort that do not require surgery and that can have no ill effects are called "noninvasive." (also see **CT Scan**)

mucous membrane: [myoo-cuss mem-brayn] The moist, thin **tissue** at the opening into the body, including the mouth, nostrils, vagina, and rectum.

N

neuro: [nyu-ro] Concerning the central nervous system (brain and spinal cord) or the peripheral nervous system (everywhere else).

neuropathy: [neur-rop-ath-ee] An inflammation or degeneration of the nerves, usually in feet, hands, arms, and legs (periphery). Symptoms often include numbness, a tingling or burning sensation, sharp pain, weakness, or even paralysis. Peripheral neuropathy is often caused by treatment **side effects** or by the HIV **virus** itself, and can usually be lessened with aggressive nutrition therapy.

night sweats: Extreme sweating during sleep to the point where the body is drenched so that the sheets and blankets need changing. Normal sweating during sleep is not a symptom of HIV.

NIH: The National Institutes of Health. The government agency that is supposed to determine the cause, prevention, and cure of diseases.

nonoxynol-9: [non-ox-i-noll nine] A spermicide (sperm-killing) chemical that also kills the **herpes** virus and protects against various STDs. It is also thought to kill HIV, and is frequently added to sexual lubricants and condoms to increase their effectiveness. Many people, however, develop an allergy to nonoxynol-9 and may experience a genital burning or itching. These people should use nonoxynol-9-free products.

O

off label: Using or prescribing a drug for a disease or condition other than those that it has been approved for. Many insurance companies and government programs will not pay for drugs unless they are prescribed for their approved purpose.

oncology: [on-coll-o-jee] The branch of medicine that studies **cancer** and tumors.

ophthalmology: [op-tha-mol-o-jee] The branch of medicine that studies and treats diseases and conditions of the eye.

opportunistic infections (OI): An opportunistic disease or infection or opportunistic **cancer** is one that people with normally healthy **immune systems** would be able to fight off. (also see AIDS; AIDS-**defining condition**; and "Chapter 7: Becoming Your Own Medical Expert")

oral hairy leukoplakia (OHL): see **leukoplakia.**

orphan drug: A drug that is not commercially profitable due to limited potential sales because it is used to treat rare diseases.

P

p24 antigen test: [P-24 Ann-tea-gin test] One of the components of the HIV **virus** is a fragment of protein called p24. This blood test measures the presence of this fragment, and therefore of the HIV **virus** itself. A positive result for p24 antigen suggests active HIV replication.

package insert: The printed instruction page or booklet included inside a package of any prescription drug or other medication. This is what the drug company wants doctors to know about their product. Because of this, it is often written in highly technical, medical terminology.

palliative: Anything that brings comfort or relief, such as painkillers, but does not actually help or cure the disease or condition.

parallel track: see **compassionate use.**

parasite: [par-a-site] Anything that lives and feeds on (or within) another living thing without extending to it any benefit in return. Humans are ideal hosts to a large number of parasite organisms (uninvited guests) such as **bacteria**, **viruses**, **fungi**, and protozoa.

pathogen: [path-o-jen] Any disease-producing **microorganism** or material, such as a toxic substance, **bacteria**, **viruses**, **fungi**, and **protozoa**.

PCP (pneumocystis carinii pneumonia): [new-moe-sis-tis car-een-ee new-moan-ya] A form of pneumonia (lung **infection**) caused by a **fungus**. An AIDS-**defining condition** that is the most common life-threatening **opportunistic infection** for people living with HIV/AIDS, and is largely preventable through drug **prophylaxis** (preventative treatment). (also see AIDS-**defining condition** and "Chapter 7: Becoming Your Own Medical Expert")

penia: [pee-nee-ya] A deficiency or lower than normal amount.

pentamidine [brand name **NebuPent®**, brand name **Pentam 300®**]: [pen-tam-eh-dine] A drug that is inhaled as vapor used for **prophylaxis** (prevention) and treatment of **PCP (pneumocystis carinii pneumonia)**.

peripheral: Pertaining to the outside edges, or occurring away from the center. Sometimes referring to the hands, arms, legs, and feet.

persistent generalized lymphadenopathy (PGL): see **lymphadenopathy**.

pharmacology: [far-ma-kol-o-jee] The branch of medicine that studies the activity of drugs in the body.

phase-I clinical trial: The first step toward FDA approval of a drug. In a phase-I clinical trial, different dose levels of a drug are tested on a small number of people to see if the drug is toxic or poisonous at these levels. Phase-I clinical trials *do not* study the effectiveness of the drug to treat a disease, only potential **side effects**.

phase-II clinical trial: The second step toward FDA approval of a drug. In a phase-II clinical trial, effectiveness and **side effects** of the drug to treat any disease is measured in some form of double-blind study on a medium-size group, usually less than a few hundred volunteers.

phase-III clinical trial: The final step toward FDA approval of a drug. A phase-III clinical trial requires as many as a few thousand volunteers, and uses some form of double-blind technique, to get the best possible information on the effectiveness and **side effects** of a drug.

PID (pelvic inflammatory disease): [pel-vick in-flam-a-tory dis-ease] A condition affecting women caused by the spread of **infection** from the vagina into the pelvic cavity. (also see AIDS-**defining condition** and "Chapter 7: Becoming Your Own Medical Expert")

placebo: [pla-see-bow] An ineffective substance (like colored water or sugar pills) that is designed to fool patients into believing that they are receiving a drug or other treatment. Placebos are often used in drug testing to compare the real effects of the active drug with the psychological effects from the patient. Many times people believe so strongly in what a treatment will do, they react as if they had the treatment, even if they only received a placebo.

plasma: [plaz-ma] The clear or light yellow liquid, basically blood without the **red blood cells**, that carries nutrition and waste products between different parts of the body. Plasma is also a key transportation medium involved with the **immune system**, and potentially may contain both disease-causing and disease-curing agents.

plasmapheresis: [plaz-ma-fer-ee-sis] The removal of whole blood, separation and removal of the **plasma** (to be used for someone else), followed by the re-injection of the remainder.

platelet: [plate-let] Cell fragments found in blood necessary for blood clotting and sealing off wounds. The number of platelets is often low in people with HIV **infection**.

pneumonia: [new-moan-ya] Pneumonia describes a number of **infections** of the lungs that can be caused by **bacteria, viruses, fungi,** or other causes. Symptoms include cough, fever, and shortness of breath. Effectiveness of treatment depends on the cause.

preclinical trial: The earliest phase of drug testing, done in a lab **in vitro** (in the test tube) and in animals, but not in humans.

presumptive diagnosis: [pre-zum-tiv die-ag-no-sis] Being diagnosed based on symptom and observation rather than actual tests, cultures, or biopsies.

Project Inform: A San Francisco–based organization which provides information about HIV/AIDS treatments and policy. (also see "Appendix B: National and Regional Resourses")

prophylaxis: [pro-fill-ax-iss] a procedure or treatment to prevent the occurrence of a disease, as opposed to eliminating a disease that already exists.

protocol: [pro-toe-call] The step-by-step outline of how a medical experiment will be conducted, including the length of the experiment, dosage levels, who may participate, and how the results will be analyzed.

pulmonary: [pull-mon-air-ee] Pertaining to the lungs.

PWA: [P W A] Person with AIDS or People with AIDS.

PWARC: A discontinued term: Person with ARC or People with ARC. (also see **ARC**)

R

randomized trial: see **double-blind trial.**

red blood cells: The red cells in the blood carry oxygen from the lungs throughout the body and remove carbon dioxide. (also see **white blood cells**)

red ribbon: The international symbol for HIV/AIDS awareness and concern, originally developed by the New York-based Visual AIDS/DIFA.

remission: [re-mish-un] The disappearance or lessening of symptoms for an extended period of time.

renal: [ree-nul] Pertaining to the kidneys.

Reoferon-A®: see **alpha interferon.**

retinitis: [ret-tin-eye-tus] Inflammation of the retina, the light sensitive layer of the eye. In people with HIV/AIDS, this is usually caused by **CMV (cytomegalovirus)**, and if left untreated, it can lead to blindness.

Retrovir®: see **AZT.**

retrovirus: A subclass of viruses that replicate themselves using an RNA template for making DNA, rather than directly using DNA as most other viruses do. HIV is a retrovirus.

risk: The likelihood that something bad will happen as a result of some action, often used as a shorthand for the "the risk of HIV transmission" for a given action or behavior. (also see "Chapter 7: Becoming Your Own Medical Expert")

S

safer sex: Any activity that can transmit HIV-infected blood, semen (cum), vaginal lubrication, or breast milk inside of another person can also transmit the HIV **virus**. The most frequent method of transmission is heterosexual (straight) and homosexual (gay) sex. The term safer sex refers to certain sexual practices (such as using a condom or other latex barrier with water-based lubricant) that greatly reduce the risk—although do not eliminate the possibility—of HIV transmission during sex.

Septra®: see **Bactrim®**.

seroconversion: [see-ro cun-ver-zhun] The time at which someone's HIV **antibody** test changes from HIV-**negative** to HIV-positive. This may be as long as six months after initial **infection**. (also see HIV-**positive**)

sero-negative: see HIV-**negative**.

sero-positive: see HIV-**positive**.

serum: [see-rum] The clear liquid, basically blood without either the red or **white blood cells**.

shingles: see **herpes zoster**.

side effects: The usually unpleasant, undesired, or negative effects of a drug other than the primary, beneficial effect. Side effects may be very minor, such as headache, skin irritation, or very major and even life-threatening.

small intestine: The portion of the gastrointestinal (GI) system which follows the stomach and empties into the **colon**. Most nutrients from food are absorbed into the body while passing through the small intestine.

spinal tap: see **lumbar puncture**.

spleen: A gland in the abdomen that is an important part of the **immune system**.

standard of care: A "standardized" outline, description, or **protocol** of what medications, treatments, and other actions "should be" taken based on certain test results or other measurable quantities. Often these outlines are oversimplified, and only take into account one or perhaps two factors.

These outlines read somewhat like a cookbook, for example, "for T-cells between 500 and 200, everyone should take AZT daily." Far from being a universal standard, each health-care professional and organization has its own unique variation, and tends to fine-tune the specific details of this "standard" every few months.

Remember, just because something is written down and widely published as being the latest and greatest "standard of care" doesn't mean that it is the right choice for you at this time.

stavudine: see d4T.

STD (sexually transmitted disease, venereal disease): A disease that is transmitted sexually, including **syphilis**, **gonorrhea**, genital **herpes**, hepatitis-B, **chlamydia**, **CMV**, genital warts, trichomoniasis, and crabs. For various technical and legal reasons, neither HIV nor AIDS are classified as an STD.

steroids: see **anabolic steroids.**

suppressor T-cells (T8-lymphocytes, CD8) One of the many types of **white blood cells** that plays an important role in the **immune system**. Once an **immune response** has been successful, the suppressor T-cells signal that the body should reduce **antibody** production and other immune responses.

symmetric: [sim-met-rick] A symptom or condition that occurs in corresponding parts of both sides of the body, for example, pain in both feet.

symptom: [simp-tum] Any observable change in a person's normal condition that indicates the presence of some disease or problem.

symptomatic: [sim-toe-matic] Experiencing the symptoms of some disease or condition. Sometimes used as a shortened form of HIV-**positive symptomatic.**

syndrome: [sin-drome] A group of specific diseases that are in some way related to a broader condition or cause.

synergy: [sin-er-jee] The interaction of two or more drugs or nutrients that work together to produce a greater effect than sum of the individual parts taken separately.

syphilis: [sif-a-lis] An STD (**sexually transmitted disease**) caused by the bacterium spirochete treponema pallidum. Penicillin is effective in treating the disease. Some believe that AIDS is in some way related to some form of drug-resistant or chronic **syphilis infections**.

T

T4 cells: see T-helper/T-suppressor ratio.

T8 cells: see T-helper/T-suppressor ratio.

T-cells (T-lymphocytes) One type of **white blood cell** that some believe to be produced in the thymus gland and which participates in various immune reactions. There are three major types of T-cells: helper, killer, and suppressor.

T-helper/T-suppressor ratio: At one time, the ratio of **T4 cells** to **T8 cells** was considered to be more meaningful than the actual values; however, many no longer consider this as meaningful.

TB: see **tuberculosis**.

thrush: see **candidiasis**.

tissue: A group of cells that acts together for a specific purpose.

TMP/SMZ: see **Bactrim®**.

toxicity (toxic side effects, toxic reaction): [tox-iss-i-tee] The extent, quality, or degree to which something is poisonous or harmful to the body. Toxic drug reactions may include **anemia**, drowsiness, fatigue, hair loss, headaches, **hives**, **kidney** failure, **liver** failure, nausea, rash, seizures, and vomiting.

toxoplasmosis: [tox-oh-plaz-moe-sis] An inflammation of the brain caused by a parasitic protozoon called *toxoplasma gondii* that is sometimes found in cat excrement and in rare meat, both of which are common sources of **infection**. About one-third of the general population is infected with *toxoplasma gondii*, but healthy **immune systems** keep this infection in check. (also see AIDS-**defining condition** and "Chapter 7: Becoming Your Own Medical Expert")

transfusion: [trans-few-zhun] The process of transferring blood, or parts of the blood (such as **serum, plasma, red blood cells,** etc.) from one person to another.

trimethoprim/sulfamethozazole: see **Bactrim®**.

tuberculosis (TB): [tube-er-cule-oh-sis] An **infection** caused by **mycobacterium tuberculosis**, usually in the lungs (pulmonary) although it may affect other parts of the body (extrapulmonary). The bacterium that causes TB can either be dormant (inactive TB) or active (active TB). Treatment consists of the administration of a combination of **antibacterial** drugs, usually for at least nine months. (also see AIDS-**defining condition** and "Chapter 7: Becoming Your Own Medical Expert")

V

vaccine: [vac-seen] A drug, taken either as a pill or by injection, that protects against a future **infection** by an organism by stimulating an **immune response**, but not disease.

Videx®: see **ddI**.

virus: [vy-russ] The smallest known infectious agent. Technically, a virus is not considered to be alive since it is unable to reproduce outside of a living host cell. A virus acts more like a toxic chemical than it does like a tiny animal. (also see "Chapter 7: Becoming Your Own Medical Expert")

W

wasting syndrome: Unexplained involuntary weight loss of more than 10 percent of the usual body weight. The actual causes may include **diarrhea**, **malabsorption**, or simply be the result of HIV **infection** itself. (also see AIDS-**defining condition** and "Chapter 7: Becoming Your Own Medical Expert")

Western Blot: The most common blood test given to determine the presence of specific **antibodies**, including HIV antibodies. The Western Blot test is very precise, meaning that it can distinguish between HIV antibodies and other antibodies. However, because it is expensive and takes many days or even weeks, it is usually used after a sample is prequalified with the **ELISA** test.

whanking: Masturbation.

white blood cells (leukocytes): [lew-co-sites] The most important part of the **immune system**, these white or colorless cells help fight disease and repair the body. Some white blood cells (leukocytes) are in a subcategory called **lymphocytes** that include T-cells and B-cells (also see **red blood cells, T-cells, B-cells**)

window period: The time between the initial **infection** of a **virus** or other **microorganism** and appearance of the first signs, symptoms, or test results indicating that disease. Once someone has become infected with the HIV virus, he or she would be able to infect others almost immediately, but that person might not test positive for HIV **antibodies** for as long as six months. (also see "Chapter 7: Becoming Your Own Medical Expert") The time between HIV infection and the point at which enough HIV antibodies are present to be measurable. This can be as short as six weeks or as long as six months. A very few people might even take as long as one year. (also see **seroconversion**)

Z

zalcitabine: see ddC.
Zerit®: see d4T.
zidovudine: see AZT.
Zovirax®: see acyclovir.

I'd like to hear your thoughts and comments about *Living Positively in a World with HIV/AIDS* and the information and resources mentioned in the appendices.

To order additional copies of this book, see your local bookstore or mail-order catalog, or contact me for more information, to place an order, or for volume discounts.

To learn about our *Living Positively* workshops, tapes, other events, and future projects, please call: (212) 924-1845 or **(800) USA-4-**HIV.

Or send your *printed* name and address to:

Mark de Solla Price
Living Positively
175 Fifth Avenue
#2359
New York, NY 10010

You may also contact me electronically via fax machine at (212)929-0822 or via the internet at 76040.3451@compuserve.com

Mark de Solla Price describes himself as "having a sexually transmitted, progressive, terminal condition . . . called *life*." He is also HIV-positive, and probably has been for over a dozen years.

As an HIV/AIDS educator and motivational speaker, Mark has been a frequent public speaker, sharing his upbeat philosophy with diverse audiences at schools, colleges, churches, and community groups on behalf of the American Red Cross, Burroughs Wellcome Pharmaceuticals, and other associations.

Mark is active in the HIV community and has worked as a peer counselor and group facilitator with a number of organizations, including New York's Healing Circle and Gay Men's Health Crisis, the world's oldest and largest HIV/AIDS service organization.

As a corporate consultant, trainer, and writer Mark has developed and conducted seminars for such clients as Harvard, Yale, NYNEX, Apple Computer, Bristol-Myers Squibb, ITT Hartford, Du Pont, and Tetra Pak.

He has advised such corporations as Time Warner, Condé Nast, Hearst, Readers Digest, CBS, GTE, Texas Instruments, Pepsi Cola, Preferred Health Care, Travelers Insurance, and even Rolling Stone.

In the early 1980s, Price studied drama with Lee

Strasberg at NYU, and later produced the off-Broadway musical (and cast album) *Tallulah*, special events, and parties at nightclubs such as Studio 54, Palladium, AREA, and others.

Mark is engaged to be married on September 3, 1995, to Vincent S. Allegrini, who owns his own hair design business in West Hartford, Connecticut. Vinny is living with AIDS and works together with Mark on a number of HIV-related projects. They love to travel and share their time between their homes in New York City and West Hartford.

Mark was born on May 17, 1960, in New Haven. His father, Derek de Solla Price (1922–1983), was Avalon Professor at Yale University, the author of six books and several hundred articles, and was an internationally renowned lecturer. His mother, Ellen de Solla Price (1925–1995), was a political activist, commentator, and artist.